The

Genius of

Flexibility

The Smart Way to Stretch and Strengthen Your Body

Bob Cooley

A Fireside Book
Published by Simon & Schuster

New York   London   Toronto   Sydney

This book is not intended as a substitute for medical recommendations by your health-care provider. Rather it is intended to offer information to help you co-operate with your choice of health-advancing experts, including alternative health-care providers, to gain optimum health. Please note that it is the ex-pressed concern of the writer that each person take responsibility for his or her health and for any and all advice received when engaging a medical or health specialist.

Resistance Flexibility Training® and The Meridian Flexibility System® are registered service marks. Use of these is prohibited without expressed written permission from the author.

FIRESIDE
Rockefeller Center
1230 Avenue of the Americas
New York, NY 10020

FIRESIDE and colophon are registered trademarks
of Simon & Schuster, Inc.

For information about special discounts for bulk purchases,
please contact Simon & Schuster Special Sales:
1-800-456-6798 or business@simonandschuster.com

Designed by Ruth Lee Mui
Photos by Michael Colarito and Bob Cooley

Manufactured in the United States of America

1   3   5   7   9   10   8   6   4   2

Library of Congress Control Number: 2005040126

ISBN-13: 978-0-7432-7087-8
ISBN-10: 0-7432-7087-8

To Pam Mitchell

Contents

PART 3: THE SIXTEEN STRETCHES

PART 4: STRETCHING FOR YOUR LIFE

The Genius Inside You

Part One

Chapter 1

My Story and Your Genius

Catapulting everything forward

ONE SPRING NIGHT IN 1976, as my friend Pam and I were walking across Boston's Commonwealth Avenue, a drunk driver in his Lincoln Continental struck us at over forty miles per hour, braking from a estimated speed of over seventy. Knocked unconscious, I was thrown twenty-five feet through the air and deposited across the intersection. My left shoulder had dislocated when I hit the pavement, and my shoulder muscles contracted so intensely that they ripped apart my upper left arm bone. My head was badly bruised, and I slipped in and out of consciousness, aware that Pam was suffering but that I was unable to help her. As I listened to the ambulance siren outside myself, inside my mind I heard these words: *"I wish myself and all others to be in life."* The next morning, I woke to the news that Pam had died within minutes after being struck.

Time stopped for me for the next two decades.

This near-death experience had a profound effect on my life. Most people who've undergone severe trauma realize afterward that something is definitely missing from their lives—something that they had always taken for granted up until that moment but could not identify or describe. It's as if you have been catapulted, in spite of yourself, into a spiritual existence but without your body. You are inexplicably stuck outside of yourself, viewing yourself and everything else from above—depersonalized. You are unable to experience your life from within your own body. Because I had been so dramatically hurled out of what was habitual and normal for myself, I had emerged with a unique kind of drive, insight, and opportunity.

I was never comfortable.
I couldn't find any position that was
ever restful or relaxing.
I was disconnected from my life,
having lost my way.
I was unable to attach to anything or anybody.
Nothing belonged to me and
I'd gladly give away anything I owned.
Many, many things just didn't make sense.

I spent the year and a half following my accident in the company of doctors. I had pulled most of the muscles in my legs, and I could not raise my left hand higher than my ear. I was deeply depressed. I went to some of the best physical therapists, orthopedic and neuromuscular specialists, sports medicine practitioners, and massage therapists in this country. Surprisingly, stretching was by far the only thing that seemed to offer help.

But I knew that the way everyone was thinking about and practicing stretching was incomplete. They had the right idea, but something really wasn't working yet. I stretched exactly as I had been instructed, but I still wasn't becoming much more flexible, and neither were the other people I observed in rehab. My expectations for recovery had not been met.

I learned from all of them, but I was not healed.
I turned to myself to discover how to heal.
I had an unquenchable passion and
insight for movement.
This, my friends told me, was my genius.

Becoming Untangled

Convinced that stretching was the right idea to heal myself, I went looking for that "secret something" about stretching that I knew had yet to be discovered. I had experimented with stretching, but like most people, I never became nearly as flexible as I wanted to be. I knew there must be some inside secret to stretching and yoga that would allow me to be as flexible as those lucky few who seemed simply to be born that way.

I had been inspired by the story of a man who was fed up with being poor. He decided to sit in a chair and stay there until he came up with an idea that would make him a millionaire. So he sat, and he sat—for days, then weeks. His unswerving determination led him to an unusual and ultimately lucrative discovery—he invented the tennis ball canister that reconditions old and dead tennis balls and brings them back to life. Out of his single-minded resolve, he found a charmingly simple solution . . . and created the life he desired. I decided to follow his lead to discover something about how muscles stretch that no one knew . . . yet!

I sat on the floor with my legs scissored wide apart. I knew that if the muscles on the inside and back of my legs stretched, then my torso and head would fold down onto the floor in front of me. I decided to do this every day for an hour, feeling and paying attention to what was happening to the muscles on the back and inside of my legs until I could somehow discover just what my muscles do when they really stretch. Like most people, I had never been even close to getting my head to the floor in front of me. Instead I found myself actually leaning backward in the opposite direction from what I intended!

For years I had tried "breathing into and relaxing" the muscles I was stretching, as taught in traditional stretching, and still the increase in range of motion was negligible. What didn't I know? Each day I returned to this position, hoping that my close scrutiny would pay off, that I would be able to identify how muscles truly stretch. I can't remember just how many consecutive days I sat on the floor waiting for some "divine intervention" to enlighten me to this

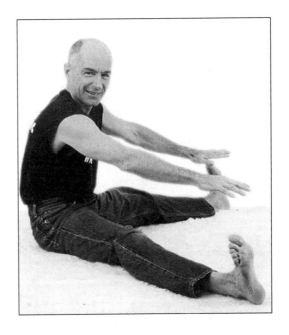

missing wisdom. Miraculously, after only a handful of days, I found the "secret" to stretching that I had been looking for.

One day, suddenly, something began to happen. Very slowly my body began to bend forward, not in tiny increments but all at once and all the way down to the floor in front of me—something I had tried unsuccessfully to do for more than twenty years. I sat back up and tried to get my torso and head to fold back down to the floor again, but with no luck. I knew that if I could only identify exactly what had happened to my muscles on the inside of my legs that allowed me to be able to bend forward to the floor, I'd then know how to repeat this miracle.

I kept waiting, for what seemed like an eternity, when suddenly my torso and head began to be pulled down to the floor again. This time I caught what was happening to

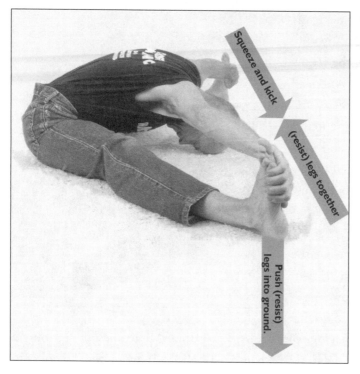

Squeeze and kick

(resist) legs together

Push (resist) legs into ground.

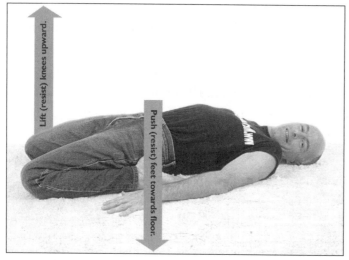

Lift (resist) knees upward.

Push (resist) feet towards floor.

inside of my legs, I felt as if they were not only elongating but also contracting. Impossible, I thought. Muscles contract only while you strengthen them. But no, I could feel the muscles *contracting*, all right. I knew they were contracting because my legs were squeezing together and pushing down against the floor—the exact opposite movements that people typically make when they are in this position and trying to stretch.

As I returned to an upright position, I decided there was only one way to know if what I had felt—muscles simultaneously contracting and stretching—was true or not. I tried another stretch. I bent my legs under me and sat on my heels, elongating the muscles on the front of my thighs. If my understanding was correct, all I had to do to get these muscles to stretch was to contract them, and then I should be able to lie backward onto

me before it slipped away. I could feel that something unique was happening inside my legs to the muscles that I was stretching, something that I didn't usually feel when I stretched.

As I paid close attention to the muscles

the floor. The way to get them to contract was by pushing my lower legs and feet against the floor. So, with an almost Promethean intensity, I began pushing.

Yes! My body started slowly to recline backward as the muscles on the front of my thighs began to stretch more. So . . . I began pushing harder and harder until I was pushing as hard as I could against the floor with my ankles and lower legs. The harder I pushed, the more my torso moved backward, until I was literally lying flat on my back on the floor. I heard these words inside my head: *You have discovered how muscles truly stretch. You must lengthen and contract them at the same time when you stretch.*

Counterintuitive, yes, and definitely startling and unbelievable. But I knew this discovery was original, new, and absolutely right. This was a completely new and different way of thinking about how to stretch. Later, I came to call this resistance stretching. Now that I knew how muscles truly stretch, I went looking to find stretches for every muscle in my body. I would squirm on the floor until I found stretches that gave me the greatest leverage for contracting the muscles I wanted to stretch. It was only later that I learned that every one of my stretch movements finished in positions that were classical hatha yoga poses. I had "rediscovered" classical hatha yoga stretches, thousands of years old.

Through continuous self-experimentation, I developed more and more stretches. Within a year and a half, I had discovered sixteen very different types of stretches for all the muscles of my body and with many varieties for each type. I also learned the necessity of stretching the muscles on the opposite side of my body before I could really stretch the muscles I wanted. Why? Simply because these other muscles needed to shorten while the ones I wanted to stretch were lengthening. I then discovered that these other muscles couldn't shorten sufficiently unless they too were flexible first. I was beginning to learn about being balanced. This was fun.

Then the "crossovers" began. Stretching started to link into affecting other aspects of myself—stretching was crossing over into affecting me physiologically, psychologically, and energetically.

Muscles, Meridians, and Personality Types

By contracting my muscles while stretching, I was continuously surprised by the increases in my flexibility. Because I now knew how to get results, I wanted more success. So I started to stretch much more regularly and intensely. I thought I could get results faster if I stretched for longer periods of time and did more repeats of the same stretch.

One day while stretching the muscles on the outside back of my thighs (my hamstrings), my bladder contracted. I asked a friend why this would happen, and she told me that in traditional Chinese medicine (TCM), the bladder meridian energy channel traverses those muscles. I stretched other specific muscles, and they too matched up with other organs and their meridians.

*My organs were being affected by
stretching specific muscles.
At first glance, the connections seemed
implausible and strange.
But they were hardly new!
These specific muscles corresponded
to meridian pathways in TCM.
The muscles, meridians, and organs
matched up exactly.*

My stretching was positively affecting my physiological health. Muscles and Energy linking meridians could be traced back to TCM—another system thousands of years old.

Another day I was stretching the muscles that twist my spine, and I found myself also being affected psychologically. I was becoming more trusting and less paranoid. I decided to see if other people could get the same psychological effects that I was experiencing. I got twenty people together (oh, my trusting friends!) to practice the same stretch for forty-five minutes. To our astonishment, everyone in the room began to behave identically. We began to speak the same, act the same, and use the same words to describe our experiences of that particular stretch. We then selected a different stretch for the next forty-five minutes. And once again, the whole room changed its personality en masse. I had to conclude from this experiment that different stretches could elicit specific ways of be-

ing—personalities, if you will. The exercises were calling forth distinct personalities inside each of us.

I wasn't just having one "eureka" moment. I was having thousands . . . and so were my friends. These moments of elucidation and discovery continually reinforced my perception that personalities and stretches matched up. The stretches were becoming conjurers calling forth distinct personality types. This ultimately evolved into my theory of the sixteen Genetic Personality Types. I call them *The Sixteen Geniuses.*

*People with the same behaviors had
the same flexibility patterns.
People with the same high personality traits
had identical muscle flexibilities.
People with the same problems had
identical muscle inflexibilities.
Identical twins had identical muscle flexibilities.
I was beginning to see Personality Types.
People are born types . . .
life circumstances modify them,
but they stay the same Personality Type.*

The Genius Breaks Through

I had learned so much! I had discovered the inside secret to stretching, meridian–muscle group associations, and the powerful ability of stretching to impact personal psychology in very predictable ways. My friends were thrilled with what I was sharing with them.

But it wasn't enough. I still didn't have my body back. That's when the best discovery occurred.

I opened a studio in Boston and began conducting research on flexibility. People came to the studio with a wide and curious assortment of requests. It was odd to me how many of the things I had discovered were also insightful and helpful to others. For example, I figured out some new stretches for muscles along my forearms and neck that a fellow stretcher felt really targeted where his tension was housed. After working on these stretches, he told me that his appendix felt better. I didn't give his observation much thought until a couple of months later, when I was hit with a really bad case of food poisoning that led to appendicitis. I used those stretches to heal my appendix (and I have kept my appendix to this day).

In the years that followed, I found that when I taught people something that was specifically valuable to them, they suddenly shared something that was specifically valuable to me. I was constantly surprised by how nonchalantly people told me the exact thing that I needed to know, at the exact moment I needed to know it. I call this the trade.

Anytime someone benefited from what I knew,
They'd offer some piece of the puzzle
*that was necessary for **my** healing.*
How did they know exactly what
I needed to know?

I was learning to heal myself
through healing others.
Intuitively we knew what the other needed.

I found good information in books and classes, but nowhere could I find what I was now experiencing through my stretching work. What I learned was emerging organically—with real people confronting real problems. Each individual problem became an opportunity to learn many things that no one knew before. People were allowing me to be their guide as I honored their authority to be their own true and unique genius—a spirited, energetic self that had countless incredible gems to teach me.

I somehow found a way to
perceive the real person,
if and only if their essence experienced
me listening to them.
I learned to listen to the voice behind the words.
The real person inside of everyone
kept telling me exactly what I needed to know.
If I argued, disconnected,
dissociated, or otherwise
diminished the value in what
they were telling me,
then they would stop speaking to me.
I was looking not at the outside person,
but at the inside person—
at their Genius.
Their Genius was healing me.
Others' Geniuses will heal you also.

People were teaching me not only subtle ways to make my stretching better but also new ways to relate, interact, and communicate. What was alien and unusual for me was as ordinary as dirt for them. I was learning how to be more fully human, to connect with parts of myself I hadn't even known existed. Things that would have been "a stretch" for me to do in the past became not just possible but surprisingly second nature. I also realized how stretching could be used positively to affect a person's past injuries, current challenges, and future aspirations.

People became translucent. It didn't matter who they were or what kind of shape they were in physically, spiritually, emotionally, or psychologically. The more I truly listened to them, soaking in much more than just their words—but their very spirit—the more everything came alive.

Twenty-five years after my accident,
I had finally returned home from my
Near-Death Experience.
I was learning what I didn't even know
I needed to know.
And I learned to trade that to others
for what I needed to know.
Their Genius was who I was looking for.
People are unbelievable.
It was just the beginning.

California Dreaming

After ten years of stretching with many incredible people in Boston, I realized I needed to catch up on my life and pursue some projects I had put on the back burner for too long. In 2000, I moved to San Jose, along with Tom Longo, my training partner at the Boston studio. There I planned to finish writing my stretching book, produce my videos, and complete a research project.

One afternoon, Tom asked me to analyze a certified Pilates instructor and advanced ashtanga yoga teacher. I worked with her, identifying which muscles were the source of her chronic pain and showing her how instantly to remove her inflexibilities in those areas. Unbeknownst to me, Olympic swimmer Dara Torres, also at the gym that day for a private Pilates session, was watching us intently from the sidelines—incredulous and amazed at the results we were having. Tom and I showed Dara and her coach how resistance stretching could make her immediately more flexible. She felt surprisingly stronger as a result.

After only five one-hour sessions, Dara went to a meet and set an American record in the freestyle! In spite of her coach's wariness, we continued to stretch Dara in preparation for competition. I stretched her for only thirty-five minutes on the following Friday, and then we stretched her for fifteen minutes before and after each race, twice in the morning and twice in the afternoon on Saturday and Sunday. At that meet she set another American record in the freestyle and won every event in which she swam—every event at her personal lifetime best times! That same evening we agreed to train her daily for the Olympics.

Dara went on to win two gold and three bronze medals at the 2000 Summer Olympics in Australia. According to Jill Lieber of *USA Today*, I had significantly helped Dara become the "Golden Girl of the Summer Games." Dara still tells everyone that flexibility training was her "secret weapon"! When the producers of *Good Morning America* approached her to appear on their "Personal Best" series, and bring with her all the equipment she had used to train herself to win, she said, "You don't need equipment. You need to talk to Bob Cooley!"

Lisa Sharkey, producer for *Good Morning America* then invited me on the show along with Dara to present the revolutionary resistance stretching to America for the first time. At the last minute, the show was relocated to a rooftop overlooking the nation's capital. (It was the day before the inauguration.) Only two one-minute segments were shown (not the four-minute sequence we had rehearsed). However, this was more than enough time to get people's attention! The Meridian Stretching Web page (www.MeridianStretching.com) received 4,500 e-mails in two days. *Good Morning America* invited Dara and me to

"I had a lot of specialists helping me in my Olympic quest, and I stretched on my own, but nothing seemed to help until I met Bob Cooley. Without the flexibility training that Bob developed for me, I could have never accomplished the five Olympic medals I had won in Sydney. . . . I know that Bob's program single-handedly developed me psychologically in very specific ways. With this mental edge, I felt personally unbelievable. There was no part of me that wasn't improved. . . . What he has figured out about stretching no one knows yet. The world will give Bob the gold."

—Dara Torres, Olympic gold medalist at age thirty-four

appear on the show again the following week. A chat line was set up for the second show. Within fifteen minutes, more than 1,000 phone calls flooded their lines. What was supposed to last twenty minutes had to be stopped after forty-five minutes. Never before did ABC have to close its chat lines due to the overwhelming volume.

The Meridian Stretching Center Web page received more than 10,000 e-mails and more than 450 phone calls within three days! Over the next year, articles appeared in *Sports Illustrated, Self, Newsweek, Outside, Elle, Oxygen, Ladies' Home Journal*, and others. We had gone public with what I had discovered. We were totally unprepared for the response. People were clamoring to learn what stretching could accomplish for them in their lives. They had clearly been waiting for this for a long time. And they were responding in droves.

The Need for More Strength and the Best Nutrition

Then, in the fall of 2002, I finally said yes to Chris Maher, an ex–Navy SEAL who had tried for six months to get me to agree to train him. After Dara's Olympic wins, I had been determined to focus on my book and not be enticed away by another athlete. He persisted, so I finally agreed to see him for a weekend of training at my house—six to eight hours per day of stretching for four days.

That was enough to get us both hooked. I couldn't resist the opportunity to demonstrate in a highly visible way the radical effect of flexibility training on the performance level and personal development of other elite athletes. Chris introduced me to Nic Bartollota, an aspiring college diver, and then to Eli Fairfield, Sean Scott, and several other professional beach volleyball partners and strength trainers. Young swimmers, gymnasts, a professional football kicker, a baseball pitcher, a marathon runner, a tennis player, a golfer, a windsurfer, a basketball player, college divers, water polo players, figure skaters, and other Olympic hopefuls chased me down to train them. Then Allan Houston, Jayson Werth, and other professional athletes came for rehabilitation and training. Sometimes we cre-

ated a complete flexibility workout for an entire athletic team.

My home on the mountaintop above San Jose on weekends looked like a professional training camp for the elite athlete or a rehabilitation center for the severely injured. I also spent that year traveling all over the country, helping many athletes as well as some severely injured people, all of whom still practice resistance flexibility training daily. This was all very exciting but exhausting.

⁓

The Olympics is about ageless dreams.
Every second counts . . . needing to
develop yourself at lightning speeds.
A focused intensity that collapses time
and creates champions.
Regular people doing extraordinary things.
Proving to everyone that they too
can accomplish miracles.
Severely injured people clinging to a hope to
come back to life better than when they left.
Intensely practicing whatever
worked so that they could
begin again to do even simple normal activities.
With discipline and dedication
that rival the mystics
they transform and inspire
everyone in their path.

⁓

But both the athletes and the very injured people pushed the envelope of my stretching knowledge. Every day they asked me to teach them more than I knew. The biggest shock came when Markus Riggleman and Steve Sierra, both certified weight and fitness trainers, pointed out that though everyone was getting incredible flexibility gains, their strength was not keeping up. Though it took a while before we listened to them, we slowly began to reverse the stretching movements to create strengthening exercises using the same muscle groups. Great! Soon all the stretches were also being used for resistance strength training.

Adding strength training also stabilized everyone's flexibility results. They kept the results longer and their flexibility became permanent.

All people who stretch, within months, quickly begin to will themselves toward the best diet possible. Their stiffness is gone and now the excess fat must go too. They start asking where they can get organic food. That means only certified organic nutrient-rich foods and wild-harvested bioavailable supplements. After eating organic food, then they want organic clothing, sheets, towels, blankets, cleaning products, and even furnishings. Everything was becoming organic.

The Genius of Flexibility

After my accident, I felt that it was totally unacceptable to have limited movement. I was completely devastated. I was extremely depressed and felt very alone and far away from everyone, including myself. I made discoveries that brought me back, way beyond just a simple physical recovery. Stretching literally transported me back into life. It gave me a stronger body than the one I had before my accident. It picked me up and repositioned me into a far better place than where I'd ever been. My perseverance in finding a solution turned my problems into gifts. My friend Bruce told me, "The scale of the trauma determined the magnitude of the gift."

Who would imagine that your particular problems could be the very guides to your success? That your problems literally light the way, like lampposts along a walkway, and that without this light you wouldn't be able to find your unique way. All the people I've met who are unbelievably successful also used their unique personal problems to develop themselves more fully, to repair and reinvent themselves, to become much more accomplished, vibrant, and alive. My car collision foreshadowed how I would find myself colliding apparent disparate databases together, like western physical therapy, traditional Chinese medicine, and psychology, and only those ideas that survived the collision would prove to be true.

Stretching makes you smile at the person who stares back at you in the mirror. It makes you curious about others. It allows you to poke fun at your ignorance and foibles. It leads you to new levels of emotional maturity, encouraging you to confide your deepest personal thoughts with the right people . . . without shame or judgment. It gives you the confidence to ask the questions you are most afraid to ask. It shows you how to be flexible all day—with yourself and with others.

⁓

And how long will it be before you admit
your genius to yourself?
Learning how to stretch exactly
the way you need to,
and in no other way,
connects you to your genius.
Catapult yourself forward.
Awaken the slumbering genius inside.
You are one in a zillion.
I believe in you.

⁓

I'd like you to try resistance stretching and experience immediate, cumulative, and permanent increases in your flexibility— and the accompanying physiological and psychological benefits. In this book I share with you what I have learned over two decades. I share with you what I've taught thousands of people about a new way to stretch that can significantly improve your body and your life. People who try resistance stretching are astounded with the results. They can't stop talking about it. They're eager to keep going, learn more, and get better results. The system I developed is a whole new way of knowing, enhancing, and enjoying your body. A lot is implied in the notion of stretching— reaching, striving, aspiring, lengthening, extending, evolving, in other words, being

more, surpassing the past in order to experience a healthy, more exceptional life.

For more than a decade, the techniques that I developed have helped thousands of people to create bodies they never dreamed of having, with physiological and psychological health benefits they wouldn't have thought were connected to improvements in their flexibility. This system has been user-tested by thousands of friends, associates, students, and clients. These stretches have proved to be invaluable to ordinary people just getting started in a fitness regimen as well as to Olympic athletes who have utilized these stretches for their flexibility and strength-training programs at their competitions.

The Meridian Flexibility System presented in this book only begins with stretching and strengthening your body. People usually start stretching to fix physical problems, but they keep stretching because of the predictable emotional, psychological, and spiritual upgrades they know they can acquire from resistance stretching.

"After three months of working in the Meridian Flexibility System, I was feeling unbelievably strong, fit, and balanced. I do not think that I could have made my fourth Olympic team without Bob's help. Thank you, Bob, for allowing me to feel and perform better than I ever thought possible."

—Eric Flaim, four-time
Olympic speed skater

The vast majority of people who try resistance stretching are not just looking for something different. They are looking for something that really works to eliminate their limitations and pain . . . not just for a few hours, but for a lifetime. Here's what people are saying about resistance stretching:

"Something the world hasn't yet seen.
Entirely new ideas and discoveries
about flexibility.
Raises the quality of your life—
and stretches your reality.
Not just extraordinary changes,
but extraordinary rates of change.

Gives me another chance,
and then another, and another . . .
I look for everyone's genius now.
It makes so much sense—it works—
the key to being flexible.
Feeling light."

Stretching teaches you that your body and your life reflect each other. Please join me as I share what I have discovered that will help you to make vast improvements in first your physical life and then your life. What you thought and felt about stretching will change forever. Many people call what I have discovered "the new way to stretch."

Chapter 2

The Inside Secret to Stretching

The discovery that will change
the way you stretch forever

WHY AREN'T PEOPLE AS FLEXIBLE AS THEY WANT TO BE? Is it that a handful of fortunate people are simply born flexible, while most of us are doomed to live the life of the Tin Man from *The Wizard of Oz*—perpetually tight, stiff, creaky, and getting worse with age? What is that secret something flexible people just naturally do when they stretch, that special knowledge that's so obvious to them yet remains a mystery to the rest of us? What's happening inside of them that is somehow not happening inside most of us?

Give Me Ten Minutes!

Give me just ten minutes. That's all I need to show you that you can be more flexible than you ever imagined. What I am about to teach you is not something you already know. It is something completely new, something that you've never been told before.

Trying something new isn't always easy. You may feel uncertain and doubtful or think that you already know what I'm about to tell you. But if you hang in there for only ten minutes, I'm confident that you will realize that what I've discovered is truly transforming. I know that after you see how much more flexible you become after trying only a few simple stretches, you are going to say, "Ahhh, that's unbelievable. A new, organic way to stretch."

Discovery exercise 1: hamstring stretch

Benefits of this stretch

Stretches the muscles on the back of your hip, thigh, lower leg, ankle, and foot.

Getting into this stretch

Lie on your back and bring your right thigh toward your chest. Then bend your right knee so that your right heel is near the back of your right hip. Your left leg can be either straight or bent.

Resisting: how to create a great stretch without pain

Grab hold of your right foot with both hands. Contract the muscles on the back of your thigh (your hamstrings) so that your heel pulls toward the back of your hips. Keep contracting your hamstrings, but simultaneously use your hands to pull your heel upward, unbending your knee and straightening out your lower leg as you lengthen your hamstrings. You are lengthening but also contracting your hamstrings at the same time. Yes, you can contract and lengthen a muscle at the same time! And yes, you must maximally contract to discover your true flexibility range. Return to the starting position and do 6–10 reps. Now change to the left leg and do the same stretch. Stand up and check out your flexibility after the complete set.

What you discover

Did you discover that you are more flexible? Most people do. Why? Because you

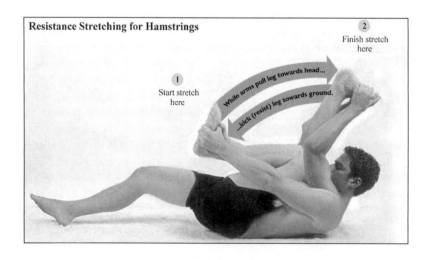

Resistance Stretching for Hamstrings

1
Start stretch here

While arms pull leg towards head...
...kick (resist) leg towards ground.

2
Finish stretch here

traditionally only lengthen a muscle to try to stretch it. But this time you lengthened *and* contracted your hamstring to stretch. You've probably never done this before. It's called resistance stretching.

The Secret Your Body Already Knows

Contracting while lengthening a muscle at the same time may seem contradictory. But in fact your body does this all the time—unconsciously and naturally. Isn't that what you do when you wake up in the morning? Don't you reach up over your head, elongating the muscles in your torso, shoulders, and arms, and then contract them at a certain point? It's natural to resist when you stretch. (And it feels good, too!)

Have you ever watched a cat get up after her nap? She reaches forward with her paws, arches her back, then pulls backward and contracts the same muscles she was trying to elongate by reaching forward. Animals instinctively understand the need to contract muscles when stretching. And they do it so well. Let's be as flexible as cats!

Resistance stretching is contracting and lengthening a muscle at the same time, something you were never told to do. You also must maximally contract while lengthening to see your true range of flexibility. This is the secret to real stretching and permanent changes in flexibility.

You know that in strength training you contract a muscle while shortening it simultaneously. But could you have guessed that in stretching you also need to contract a muscle while lengthening it at the same time? The harder you contract a muscle when stretching—by pushing or squeezing some part of your body against the floor, a wall, yourself, or someone else—the more your flexibility will improve. It may surprise you to learn that your muscles need to contract in both strength training and in stretching. And that it takes twice the force to stretch a muscle than to strengthen it!

Get Immediate Results

All right, now let's really go somewhere with stretching! Let's use resistance stretching for your lower body involving the muscles on the front of your thighs (your quads) and then for your upper body involving muscles on the back of your shoulders (your trapezius). You'll also learn how you can change each stretch into a strengthening exercise for the same muscles.

Remember: In resistance stretching, you always start in a position where the muscles you want to stretch are shortened as much as possible. And then to stretch these muscles, you contract and lengthen them at the same time by moving some part of your body. The process of contracting and lengthening a muscle at the same time causes those muscles to stretch in a new and powerful way.

Once you see how the resistance stretching technique works, you'll discover you can become as flexible as you wish ▮where in your body. I'll show you how to choose the stretches for the parts of your body you want to make more flexible. You'll do several reps of the chosen stretches, noticing a remarkable increase in flexibility after each stretch. It's fun to have other people watch you while you do these stretches. They can observe how much more flexible you look, while you can observe how much more flexible you feel.

You pull yourself together when you use resistance stretching, instead of yanking yourself apart as you do in traditional stretching.

Discovery exercise 2: front of thigh stretch at wall

Benefits of this stretch

Stretches the muscles along the front of your hip, thigh, lower leg, ankle, and foot.

Getting into this stretch

Kneel on all fours with the wall directly behind you. Bend your left knee and bring your left leg up against the wall, resting the top of your foot against the wall (you can use a towel or small pillow to protect your foot). Step up onto your right foot, lunge deeply forward, and slant your torso slightly forward.

Resisting: how to get a stretch without pain

While leaning forward in a lunge, push against the wall with your left foot by contracting the muscles on the front of your left thigh. As you continue to push your left leg and foot against the wall, bring your hips back to your foot against the wall by pushing yourself forward with your right leg. Moving your body backward lengthens the muscles on the front of your thigh, but because they are also contracting, they stretch. That's right! You're getting it!

Remember, the same muscles that are being stretched are being contracted. Stretching and contracting a muscle are not

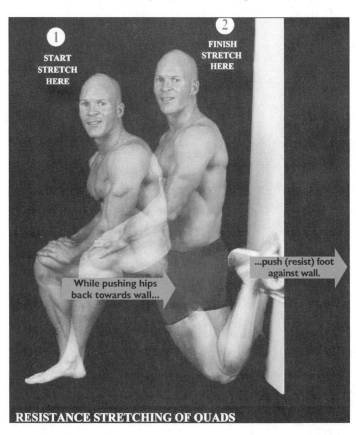

① START STRETCH HERE

② FINISH STRETCH HERE

While pushing hips back towards wall...

...push (resist) foot against wall.

RESISTANCE STRETCHING OF QUADS

mutually exclusive endeavors. And you must maximally contract while lengthening to see your true flexibility range. They work together to create the most powerful stretches possible.

What you discover

This use of resistance results in greater flexibility—muscles begin to stretch farther than before. In principle, to generate great resistance in any stretch, you need to oppose or fight against the stretch, so to speak.

Now you are learning how to resist in a stretch by feeling how your body naturally does it. You absolutely need to resist maximally sometimes in order to make any muscle really flexible.

After resisting only once, you should be able to bend your knee farther and get your ankle closer to the back of your hips: instant flexibility! After repeating the stretch 6–10 times, you'll notice even greater increases in your muscle's elasticity.

Let's add strengthening now.

Don't stop with stretching—strengthen the same muscles. Switch sides. You can strengthen your quads by starting in the position where you finished your stretch, where the muscles are as long as possible. Continue to contract your quads by pushing

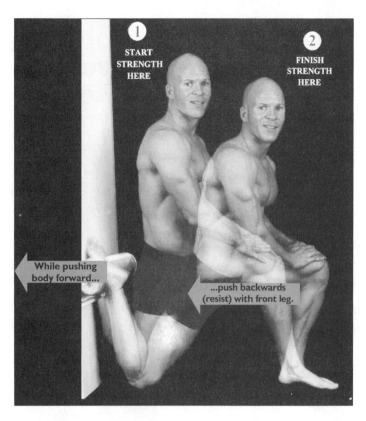

①
START
STRENGTH
HERE

②
FINISH
STRENGTH
HERE

While pushing body forward...

...push backwards (resist) with front leg.

against the wall with your ankle and foot, as you push yourself forward into a lunge. Resist your forward lunging by pushing yourself backward with your front leg. That's how you strengthen your quads. You need to use maximum force here also.

To reverse any stretch into a strengthening exercise, simply reverse the starting and ending positions, and reverse how you create resistance—but in both cases always keep contracting the muscles you are stretching or strengthening.

Let's try a stretching exercise for your upper body now.

Discovery exercise 3: grapevine arms

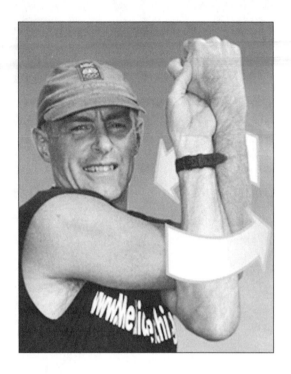

Benefits of the stretch (and strengthening)

Stretches the muscles on the back of your shoulders, neck, arm, and index finger.

Getting into this stretch

This stretch can be done standing, sitting, or lying on your back—whatever feels most comfortable to you. Cross your arms, twist your lower arms around each other, and clasp your hands together. This lengthens muscles on the back of your shoulders and down your arms into your index finger.

Resisting: how to create a stretch without pain

Press and twist your arms against each other by pulling your elbows against each other and pressing your hands together. This causes the muscles on the back of your shoulders and arms that have been lengthened to contract and stretch. You can tilt and turn your head to either side to create more stretch in your neck. Keep resisting for 6–10 seconds, then switch sides. Remember to maximally resist in order to see your true flexibility range.

What you discover

As unbelievable as it may seem, using resistance gives you immediate changes in flexibility. You'll find that the increases in your flexibility accumulate and eventu-

ally become permanent. Repeat the three stretches in this chapter. They should feel a lot different during and after the second and third sets—repeats of the exercises. You experience immediate changes in flexibility and strength after just a few exercises using resistance stretching (and strengthening).

What's Next?

There's a lot more to resistance stretching than simply contracting and stretching a muscle simultaneously. This kind of stretch opens the door to a whole new way of thinking about your body. As you learn more and begin to experience what is available to you through resistance stretching and strengthening, you can create a whole new way of being.

Chapter 3

Stretching Myths and Realities

Changing your beliefs about stretching

IF YOU'RE LIKE MOST PEOPLE, you've probably already tried several forms of stretching and yoga. Common assumptions everyone has about stretching often go unquestioned.

You may believe that some people are just born naturally flexible. You may assume that if someone is flexible physically, then he is also mentally flexible. You might assume that stretching is a form of passive exercise and that it won't give you the rigorous workout you're looking for. You might believe that men are less flexible than women and children more flexible than adults. You may think stretching is a warm-up, something you do before the "real" exercise begins. You may have concluded that stretching is a waste of time because you didn't notice much of an increase in your flexibility or experience other benefits from it in the past. You might have exacerbated old injuries by stretching, or even created new ones. You have never experienced stretching as an activity that can impact all other areas of your life, not just your physical body. These are all false beliefs.

Resistance stretching advances every aspect of your life. In the process, many of your firmly held beliefs about stretching will change. The following ten principles of resistance stretching ask you to rethink many of your ideas or beliefs about stretching. These ten principles are not just theory. They were derived from my experience with thousands of people.

A New Way to Stretch

1. You need to contract and lengthen your muscles while stretching.

Placing yourself in overextended positions is not stretching. Pulling and yanking on your muscles is not stretching. When you stretch a muscle, it naturally contracts and resists to produce the stretch. Your true flexibility range occurs only when you maximally resist while lengthening. It takes twice the tension to stretch a muscle as to strengthen it! Contracting a muscle while simultaneously stretching it is called resistance stretching.

2. Resistance stretching offers immediate, cumulative, and permanent increases in flexibility (and strength).

Most people never become as flexible as they want to be, but not because there is something inherently wrong with them or they're not athletic enough. They aren't achieving their flexibility goals because they haven't added resistance to the stretching equation. By resisting the stretch, necessary tension is created in the muscle, which results in an immediate increase in flexibility. Maximally resisting brings exceptional increases. Getting into a stretch position is not enough to get a true stretch. You must add resistance! Because a muscle must contract when you stretch it, that muscle must also be strong enough to produce the stretch. Reversing the direction and appli-

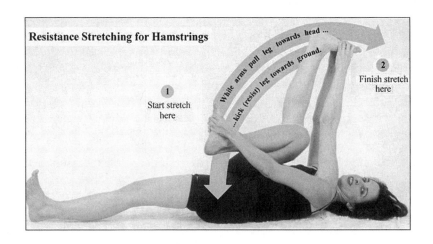

Resistance Stretching for Hamstrings

While arms pull leg towards head ...

...kick (resist) leg towards ground.

1
Start stretch
here

2
Finish stretch
here

cation of resistance of any stretch movement changes that exercise into a strength-training exercise. Thus sufficient strength is a necessity when stretching.

3. Resistance stretching takes the pain out of stretching and protects you from injuring yourself from overstretching.

Many people have abandoned stretching because they felt they weren't getting the results they wanted or because their stretching led to injury or unreasonable soreness. Only by contracting your muscles when you stretch does stretching finally become pleasant rather than painful. Better yet, your muscles are protected from over-stretching. Stretching without contracting a muscle produces a false range of motion, known as substitution, and ultimately results in overstretching and injury. You must stretch the balancing muscle to ensure a successful stretch. Resistance stretching takes the unnecessary risk out of stretching.

4. Stretching is one of the most effective self-help preventive medicines.

Individual stretches have often been reported to improve specific physiological and psychological conditions, allowing individuals to choose exact stretches that help them heal chronic problems and replace dysfunction with healthy functioning. Phys-

ical, spiritual, emotional, and psychological benefits from stretching provide powerful motivation for practicing stretching regularly. Stretching accelerates the rate of personal change.

5. To achieve the highest level of improvement in flexibility, it is essential that other people assist you.

Many things can be done only by yourself—no one else can do them for you. Unquestionably you can acquire incredible increases in your flexibility by stretching on your own, but more significant gains require people to help you stretch. This is because when another person assists you, you can resist him or her with your greatest amount of resistance—greater contractions than you

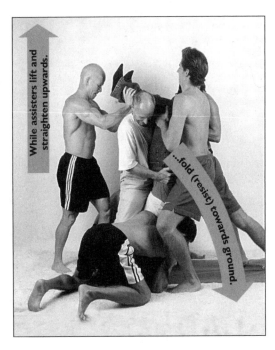

While assisters lift and straighten upwards.

...fold (resist) towards ground.

can generate when resisting against yourself. Maximum resistance brings maximal results.

6. Natural breathing produces the best stretching results.

To get maximum benefits from stretching, you must be open to new ways of breathing. Each type of stretch produces different ways of breathing, creating tension and relaxation. Ingrained patterns of breathing are broken down and replaced with new, healthier breathing habits. As your breathing improves, you will achieve greater ranges of motion. In stretching, you go looking for the pain and tension in your body in order to remove it. This can happen only by not controlling the way you breathe. Natural breathing makes everything feel effortless.

7. Everyone has unique patterns of flexibility, and everyone can be flexible.

Flexibility is an equal-opportunity endeavor! Everyone can be flexible, regardless of gender, race, or age. Just because you are tight in one place does not mean that you are tight everywhere. Just because you appear physically flexible does not mean you are equally flexible spiritually, emotionally, and psychologically. Different personality types have predictable flexibility patterns. Positive and negative life conditions affect your flexibility. Regular stretching is positive conditioning.

8. Stretching affects every type of tissue in your body.

Each stretch presented in this book improves the health of a different type of tissue, including muscles, fascia, tendons, ligaments, joint capsules, cartilage, bones, circulatory and lymphatic flow, oxygenation of blood, endocrine functions, cerebrospinal fluid, and so on. Some parts of your body require more time to become flexible than other parts because of the nature of those tissues. For example, your hamstrings take more time to make flexible than your quads.

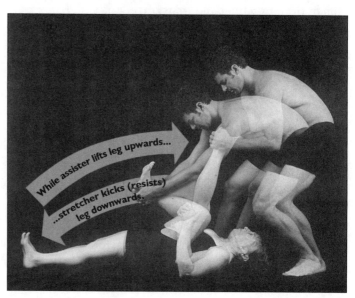

While assister lifts leg upwards...

...stretcher kicks (resists) leg downwards.

9. Stretching involves using intense force for dramatic increases in strength, power, speed, and accuracy.

Stretching matches and often exceeds all other forms of exercise in intensity and use of force. When you stretch a muscle, twice the tension is generated in the muscle compared to when you strengthen the muscle. In other words, it takes twice the force to stretch a muscle than to strengthen it. Maximal resistance must be attempted regularly when stretching to reach maximal flexibility. Because a muscle's ability to shorten is directly determined by its flexibility, as your muscles gain flexibility you can expect an immediate 15–20 percent increase in strength—without any additional weight training—as well as significant gains in power, speed, and accuracy. Remember, all stretch movements can become strength-training exercises simply by reversing the direction of the movement. You need sufficient strength to contract your muscles maximally when stretching them.

10. Nothing is a substitute for stretching.

Within minutes after stretching, *everyone* feels better. There is something inherently healing and pleasurable about stretching. Stretching teaches you how to handle the most intense situations. The stretching pro-

grams presented in Chapters 9–13 provide sixteen different types of stretches at four distinct levels. Therefore, there are types of stretches to target your specific physiological and psychological concerns.

Few other activities bring you such life.
Stretching is timeless—it gets better with age.
In the near future, it will be very hard to find
anyone who doesn't stretch.
Let stretching connect you to your genius.

I hope you're beginning to think differently about stretching—about how it works and what it can do.

Mastery

Learning the 10,000 things about any one thing

Mastery is one of those life experiences that is difficult to capture in words. It's not about winning medals or being "the best" in any competitive sense. It has nothing to do with innate talent or gifts. Mastery explicitly refers to a mental development—establishing an unshakable mental prowess. When you decide to master something that compels and fascinates you, your journey might look something like this:

You'll discover that your mind directs you to pay attention to what exactly you need to learn. Unbeknownst to many, you do not get to decide what you are going to pay attention to; instead, you are supposed to *be* where your attention is, and this allows your mind to collect the information it needs in order for you to learn. Though your mind leads the way, you learn to defer to your body to show you how to do what you're thinking. Don't let your thoughts, no matter how great they appear, distract you from following your body's way of doing things. You'll learn to not hold on to past feelings or sensations that you've experienced, no matter how phantasmagoric they were. Instead you will reexperience them every day as you practice when you follow your attention.

You are in mastery mode.
Three years of being this way brings you to
mastery.

As your focus continues to take in the ever-widening "field" of possible things to pay attention to, you begin to funnel toward your goal. Though your "fishing net," or field of possible things to pay attention to, needs to stay open and be ever increasing, your mind will funnel toward the target. You arrive in the "zone"—self-actualizing. While this is occurring the speed of your comprehension gives the impression of expanding time, where each moment feels like days or even many years are passing. Day after day new insights—little jewels of wisdom—will come to light until you have

literally learned thousands of things. Soon you will get it. Your collected experiences are like the rungs of a ladder that lift you to mastery.

In Western science it is known that it takes approximately 10,000 molecules to pass across a cell's membrane before communication from one cell to another reaches threshold. It's not a coincidence that the Chinese believe there are 10,000 things you need to know before mastery occurs. I believe this to be true when anyone follows their passion and their genius to complete their masterpiece of living.

Stretching mastery is well within anyone's reach. You can create your own stretching opus. In the process of reaching mastery everyone I know defines his or her own sovereignty and authority. They develop unswerving trust in themselves and their own capacity to solve problems and pursue new possibilities. They command tremendous respect and yet are light and approachable in their manner.

Mastery gave me a mantra I now carry with me everywhere:

"Thank you for telling me that," I say, in reply to every one of the 10,000 questions I ask about everything!

The next chapter outlines the benefits of stretching (physiological, spiritual, emotional, and psychological). Prepare to be astonished!

Chapter 4

The Benefits of Being Flexible

Help yourself

MOST LIKELY YOUR PARENTS NEVER STRETCHED. If they did, they probably gave up in short order. And who can blame them? The old way of stretching yanked their muscles apart, felt more like a chore than a pleasure and, to add insult to injury, usually produced few or no real benefits.

Resistance stretching isn't like that tired piece of exercise equipment you retired to the basement because you got bored with it. Resistance stretching is fun. It feels good. And it takes minutes, not months, to see visible, positive changes. It's infectious and inspiring. And soon it will become a life passion for you.

Everyone who has tried resistance stretching continues with it. They *never* stop. They continue not only because they see immediate improvements in their flexibility, but also because, as time goes on, they discover other benefits that come from feeling, looking, and behaving like the person they were intended to be.

People who have stretched for a while know that changes from stretching are predictable and self-prescriptive—they can decide what they want to work on, do those stretches, and reap the benefits they desire. The predictable changes and self-actualizations from stretching are the hallmark of the Meridian Flexibility System.

The Physical Benefits of Stretching

Astounding physical and physiological changes result from developing greater flexibility. As your flexibility increases, you'll experience more fluidity in your movements. Suddenly you are sitting up straighter, walking taller, feeling lighter, and becoming more youthful and childlike in your movements. Your power, strength, and endurance skyrocket. Chronic pain disappears. Your diet improves, future injuries don't have a chance, and your general health is enhanced. You feel stronger, more resilient, and vigorous. You are mystified by your emerging physical prowess.

Flexibility turns your anger and hatred into love

As you engage in conflict with your own body while stretching, you are learning to transfer these skills when engaging in conflict with others and turning problems in relationships into deeper love. As the chronic discomfort in your body leaves, the angst about survival diminishes.

Flexibility wakes you up and shows you how to live in the present

As you remove habitual patterns of discomfort in your body, you find yourself waking up as if from a deep sleep. By focusing your attention on stretching, you find yourself living more in the present. Your physical instincts improve—survival instincts come to the fore, and you find yourself better able to set boundaries and limits with other people.

Flexibility determines how well you move and improves your posture

Your flexibility absolutely determines what movements you are able to make and how fast, accurate, and powerful those movements can be. That box on the top shelf suddenly becomes more reachable. Your posture naturally becomes upright without any need for mental reminders to sit up straight or stop slouching. Your biomechanical efficiency has been upgraded.

Flexibility harnesses your strength, power, and endurance

The ability of any muscle to shorten is directly controlled by its ability to lengthen. By increasing your flexibility, your muscles are able to shorten and contract maximally, which translates into increased power, speed, and acceleration.

Flexibility relieves pain, prevents injuries, and promotes comfortable living

Many chronic as well as acute myofascial pains are the direct result of muscle shortness. Increase the length of your muscles, and watch your back, knee, elbow, and other pains disappear. Increases in flexibility and strength also help to prevent future injuries.

Flexibility heals and overhauls your physiological health

A flexibility perk is that your internal health improves—and in very specific and predictable ways. These stretches have helped thousands of people make specific health improvements. With the information presented in this book, you can individualize your own stretching program based on your unique needs.

Flexibility results in improved diet

No matter what diet you think is the best for you, everyone who stretches regularly finds that his eating habits improve. Organic foods find their way onto your plate and suddenly become more attractive than anything else. Nutrient-rich foods replace empty foods.

Flexibility creates athletic prowess

It should be no surprise to you from what you have already read about athletes who have won gold medals at the Olympics (and who credit a big part of their success to resistance flexibility training) that flexibility is the foundation to all physical exercise. Strength, aerobic, and skill performance all depend on flexibility.

Flexibility teaches you to rest and handle stress and distress

When you know how to rest, you can build a better you because your body rebuilds itself during rest. Stretching teaches you how to embrace appropriate amounts of rest to remove undesirable stress and distress.

Flexibility teaches you how to protect and defend yourself instead of being defensive yourself

There are many ways to defend yourself and to keep good boundaries, and stretching leads the way. Learn that there is also no need to defend yourself if you are not being attacked.

Flexibility makes you more youthful and solid

Everyone who stretches regularly gets younger and better looking. Not only will you move and feel like a person with a much younger body, but you'll also have a new tool at your disposal to modify and adjust your body so those aches and pains from aging become less intrusive or even disappear. People who aren't stretching are aging prematurely.

The Spiritual Benefits of Stretching

Unbelievable spiritual changes result from developing greater flexibility. Becoming more flexible connects you with positive life changes while it disconnects you from objectionable parts of your life. Changes in awareness and modifications in perspective become daily occurrences. You can directly experience the wonderful connection between your body and your life from stretching. You find yourself making better choices, showing greater integrity, and enjoying doing the things that are good for you. You begin to live more and suffer less, experiencing everything about energy and spirit, living timelessly.

Flexibility moves you from doing things that aren't good for you to holding higher values

Stretching pushes your values toward humanitarian concerns. You find yourself becoming more ethical, forthright, principled, and empathetic.

Flexibility turns resistance into yielding

You find yourself becoming less resistant to positive life changes—learning to open yourself to embrace the good—and more resistant to negative influences and desires.

Flexibility is a reflection of your life

Every tension in your body is a reflection of how you live your life. You discover that the joys and problems of the world are also reflected in your body. Stretching allows you to experience the interconnections and the oneness to life and to powers greater than yourself.

Flexibility opens you to new awareness and perspectives

Becoming more objective, viewing others and yourself from "above" are trademarks of stretching. Learn to view others and yourself from both inside and outside yourself—balance your perspective.

Flexibility teaches you about timelessness—simply living

No rat race here, just days and days of your life. Becoming filled with life. Viewing everything with a relative time reference—the past, future, and present are all happening now.

Flexibility can connect you to a power greater than yourself

Learn about spirituality from your body. Become more empathetic, open, and fair-minded, and dismantle your false beliefs. Become more serene, calm, still, and peaceful. Stay connected by resolving conflicts. Learn to embrace all world philosophies and religious wisdom.

Flexibility shows you how to enjoy rather than suffer through life

As you become more flexible, your spiritual energy is unleashed. You find yourself getting up early, stretching, eating well, exercising throughout the day, playing at work, and losing track of time because you are reveling in life, enjoying everything moment by moment. Flexibility teaches you to escape the bondage of the clock. It gets you out of your head and turns off the internal noise.

Flexibility lets you be in your body and to enjoy being there

You can now feel specific parts of your physical body that you used to feel disconnected from. You learn how to stay connected with your physical body.

Flexibility teaches you about being serene, calm, still, and peaceful

There's no place like home, and it begins within. Bring inner peace outward. People are on the same planet because they need each other.

Flexibility turns everyone into a seeker of illumination

It happens almost unnoticed at first. But soon everything is about energy and light. Energy and imagination are linking you into the transcendental.

Flexibility results in sweeping changes and transformations in every aspect of oneself and one's life

The whole world is currently going through the largest evolutionary shift ever. Be in on the changes.

The Emotional Benefits of Stretching

Exciting emotional changes result from developing greater flexibility. Dismantling the emotional armor we wrap about ourselves is a principal benefit of flexibility. You find yourself maturing emotionally—becoming more intimate, more attached, more sensitively engaged in other people's lives. All sorts of things begin to look and work better—your self-image, your confidence, and your appearance. The things you really like and need suddenly are made clear to you. You free yourself from the traumas of the past and learn how not to repeat the same mistakes. Despondency and anxiety loosen their grip, and in their place emerge burgeoning and intensely exciting and fulfilling creativity and passion.

Flexibility turns anxiety into excitement

Becoming more flexible instantly turns chronic dread and anxieties into eager anticipations. Motivations soar and gratification increases.

Flexibility shows you how to be more conscious of what you truly desire

Increasing your flexibility makes you more conscious of what you truly desire, shedding false illusions about attractions and attachments.

Flexibility shows you how to free yourself from the past— and learn from it

Benefiting from the past mistakes of others and yourself, and finally getting the nurturing you need, is what stretching is all about.

Flexibility teaches you to respond retroactively

You learn to process, sometimes for days, previous events as you move into clarity about yourself and others.

Flexibility teaches you new ways to breathe

Every stretch you do brings you to a new position in life. In every new situation, you are asked to breathe differently. New ways of breathing literally morph your physical body. Breathing elevates your mood and affects your feelings of self-worth and self-esteem.

Flexibility shows you how to relax naturally and to use tension appropriately

As you learn to resist maximally when stretching, your body naturally employs greater levels of tension while simultaneously relaxing you. It takes unimaginable levels of tension to perform skilled movements, and only by being emotional can this happen.

Flexibility brings up your good looks, beauty, image, and likableness

Everyone wants to put forth his or her best face and body. Because stretching centers you emotionally and helps you to understand who you are from the inside, you light up on the outside, glowing. Remove your tensions and you find that you like yourself more.

Flexibility shows you how to be more free, caring, honest, and creative

Different stretches develop your ability to have more freedom, to better care for yourself and others, to risk the embarrassment of being more honest, and to access inner reservoirs of creativity.

Flexibility teaches you to be more social and enjoy yourself socially

Social anxieties turn into social skills, as you move successfully through the social maze. Learn to return the attention that others give you by giving back to them.

Flexibility increases positive self-affirmations

Uplift yourself and others by affirming what is important. Hear yourself say the nicest things about yourself.

Flexibility increases your self-esteem, self-worth, and self-respect

If you don't have enough of any of these, you develop more—and even have enough left over to give to others.

Flexibility teaches you how to be fulfilled sexually

Only by being emotionally available can you have satisfying sexual relationships. Mature emotionally into relationships that bring ultimate satisfaction.

Flexibility teaches you team spirit at home, in business, and in prayer

Groups of people can do what individuals cannot. Teamwork reflects what the people want and helps the groups to manifest the needs of many.

The Psychological Benefits of Stretching

Cathartic psychological changes result from developing greater flexibility. Stretching allows you to experience highly desirable personality or behavioral traits that quickly become integrated into your self. It makes you more psychologically "fit"—better at decision making, more self-expressive, and more trusting. You think with greater clarity, become more focused and articulate, and have a perspective that is forward looking and future minded.

Flexibility turns fear into knowledge

Working on your body and learning how to overcome the fears you have associated with this is a model for handling other fears in life.

Flexibility shows you how to be clear and future minded

Being flexible about your own areas of ignorance is your bridge to knowledge. Stretching helps you to aspire to greater levels of understanding, clarity, and humor.

Flexibility develops sixteen high personality traits

Sixteen of the best personality qualities can be developed from stretching. Turn every negative trait into its opposite high trait.

Flexibility teaches you about mastery and mental prowess

Learn aristocratic ways of being civil, well mannered, and authoritative. Become more understanding, trusting, decisive, and expressive. Being more flexible shows you how to speculate, analyze, prove things, debate, and research. Become a great problem solver.

Flexibility teaches you how to be detached and sympathetic, and also how to problem-solve

Being attached to others is essential, but that doesn't mean you can't also be detached and thoughtful, helping to analyze their situations and make good decisions—for others and yourself.

Flexibility teaches you to be sober, self-expressive, and forceful

Being unafraid to be with people we like and are attracted to, using the right words to say what we mean, and being able to stand behind what we say can all be learned from stretching—this is sobriety.

I found that flexibility increases my courage, dismantles my grief, keeps me in good spirits, and increases my ability to love. Stretching is fast becoming one of the best preventive medicines. In the near future, it will be very hard to find anyone who does not stretch.

We'd love to hear some of the ways stretching has benefited your life. Log on to our Web site and e-mail us your stretcher's story. We can't get enough of these!
www.MeridianStretching.com

A New
Essential
Flexibility

Part Two

Chapter 5

Psychological Self-Education and New Ways of Breathing

How to create psychological and emotional well-being

IT'S WONDERFUL WHEN we accomplish something effortlessly, when we move eloquently, without thinking too much or too hard about what we are doing or how we are doing it. If you've ever played tennis, you've probably experienced what it's like to get into the rhythm of your service game. It's beyond words, really—from the moment you toss the ball above you, you move with a streamlined ease and economy. Your body is showing you how to serve. But the moment you begin to overthink it, or try to control your arm movement too much, or become apprehensive about hurting some part of yourself when you move, then your fun is dampened and you begin to chock. The racket starts to feel microscopic and the ball seems cursed.

If for some reason your arm doesn't move correctly when you serve, all the thinking in the world won't ever change it. If you already know the correct way your arm should move, then you and your mind already know. The knowledge is literally at your fingertips. It's your body that can't do it yet, not your mind.

You need to stretch the necessary muscles so that they can contract and execute the correct ideas about serving. Once flexible, your body serves the ball naturally and correctly, and your mind is in the zone.

Any unresolved past injury can stop this natural flow from occurring. You'd like so much not to be so tentative, you want to be able to put everything you've got into the task at hand, without having to think about it. Your mind needs to be free. Stretching can release you from the mental chains that bind you, so that you can begin to move again as you did when you were a child, without the intrusive interference of your mind. Let's see how to get your body and your mind on the same side.

Taking Inventory Versus Controlling Your Attention

Many meditative and contemplation techniques instruct you to place your attention on something inside or outside of yourself and keep it there. You are encouraged to avoid any distraction and to select a solitary point of concentration that you return to again and again. You do not allow your mind to wander, and if it does, you bring it back to a state of alert attention to that single reference point.

This is *not* what happens in resistance stretching. I found that when I acknowledge what I am aware of, and don't shrink from it, I learn a lot more about myself and others. I

prefer to let myself take inventory of everything that my mind seems to direct me to pay attention to when I stretch. I learn how to stretch at a very fast rate when I do this. When I control my attention, it seems to impede my growth and slow my learning.

You already know that when you stretch, there's a "body rule" that you follow: Allow your body to teach you how it wants you to move. A similar rule applies to your mind. You decide what stretch you want to do but not where to put your attention. Once you decide to do a particular stretch, your mind directs your attention to whatever it is you need to learn. It's your job to be where your attention goes and not try to control its wanderings. In this way you are observing the world both inside and outside of yourself. I call this "free-attentional focus."

As you stretch, don't edit anything you find yourself paying attention to, even if it seems frivolous or silly. If you try to constrain or tame your thoughts, feelings, memories, or sensations, you will miss out on the important psychological impacts of stretching.

Free-Attentional Focus Calisthenics

To get yourself accustomed to engaging yourself psychologically as you stretch, let's try a short exercise in free-attentional focus, using a simple torso and arm side stretch (called a #2 lateral bend stretch in the stretching routines).

Stand with your feet a little wider than your shoulders (see photo below). Bring your arms above your head and grasp one hand just below the other hand. Laterally bend to one side. As you straighten back up to center, resist yourself by pulling yourself sideways (as if someone is pushing you from the side as you resist against him to return to center).

What were you aware of as you did this stretch? Repeat the stretch on both sides several times, taking careful note of your thoughts and emotions. Here are a few questions to help get you started:

- Did you feel the sides of your torso stretch?
- Were you looking up at your hand or at the ceiling?

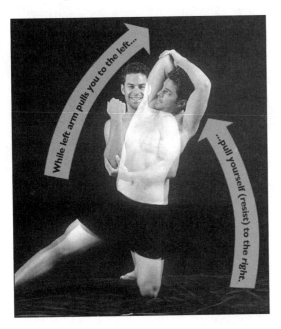

While left arm pulls you to the left...

...pull yourself (resist) to the right.

- Did the stretch bring up anything from your past?
- What determined how many reps you attempted?
- Were you thinking about anything in particular?
- Was your vision affected by doing the stretch?
- Were you aware of your liver?
- Were you aware of being anxious or excited?
- Did you like or dislike doing the stretch?
- Were you aware of your tendons?
- Would you prefer practicing this stretch with others?
- Did this stretch improve your looks in a particular way?

I'm sure as you did this exercise you were aware of some of these things and not others. And you probably thought of a few questions that I didn't think to ask. The point is that each person becomes conscious of different sensations, memories, issues, longings, and so on at different times when he or she does this or any stretch. It is very important to note all of these thoughts, no matter how insignificant or inappropriate they seem. Later, you'll identify what specific stretches can accomplish for you mentally as you begin to share your stretching experiences with others and confirm similar psychological changes for each type of stretch.

What Actually Happens Psychologically When You Stretch?

As you free yourself to notice the subtle changes that occur when you do a particular stretch, you are learning about the mental part of stretching. You cannot observe these changes if you are habitually trying to control what you pay attention to. It doesn't matter if you think your foot should be corrected, or that you should be resisting in a particular way. What matters is where your attention is at that specific moment, not what you think you should pay attention to.

You are learning very different ways of being when you stretch. These changes in your perception of yourself and what's happening around you collectively define the characteristic way of being of one of sixteen personality types I identify. What actually happens as you stretch is that you begin to experience very positive high personality qualities while simultaneously dismantling the opposite low psychological qualities. Sounds good, huh? These personality qualities are associated with the sixteen genetic personality types.

Give Yourself Another Chance

As you practice a stretch repeatedly, you begin to act, think, and feel differently. Basically, you are learning to be in all the ways you've witnessed other people being but that seemed to elude you. Flexibility allows us to be more adaptable, to accommodate ourselves to new circumstances, improving our chances of survival and growth. Unlike a machine that functions according to simple cause and effect, humans learn through interdependent feedback loops, constantly renewing and recycling.

Our physical bodies do this all the time. The pancreas, for instance, replaces most of its cells every twenty-four hours. Our stomach lining replaces itself every three days. Our white blood cells are renewed every ten days. And so on. This capacity for self-renewal allows us to reach creatively beyond physical and psychological boundaries, to learn, develop, and improve.

We all have aspects of our personalities that we'd like to bring "up"—we want to be more self-expressive, or more empathetic, or more assertive or helpful. We all also have aspects of ourselves we dislike, are ashamed of, or are secretive about. The key to stretching is to turn a flashlight on the positive parts of yourself by selecting the specific stretches that reveal to you how to be in those specific ways while reversing their opposite negative traits (the parts you'd like to leave behind). Stretching literally turns past traumas into triumphs.

Each stretch develops you in very specific ways physically, and also psychologically. I call this learning "new ways of being." To give you a taste of what you might experience psychologically from resistance stretching, let's first look at the general characteristics of the four personality groups.

The Four Personality Groups

I am certainly not the first person to uncover a psychology of personality. A great diversity of thinkers, from Jung to Erikson to Ichazo, have supported the notion that people fall into certain personality type categories and that within these categories are specific areas of commonality. These common characteristics might originate from any number of measurable criteria—traits, ego states, physiognomy, disorders, behaviors, sexual motivations, genes, even the shape of the skull. All of these theories are fascinating, and many can provide valuable insight into our knowledge of how a personality is formed and develops over time.

But my own particular ideas on personality types derived from my experiences with stretching and how different stretches affected me and the thousands of people I have worked with. These ideas evolved organically and spontaneously out of many people's experiences with specific stretches and what we began to observe in ourselves as we delved more deeply and intensely into the different stretches. I had even gone so far as to test identical twins who were separated at birth, thinking that if personality types were genetic, then regardless of how the twins were conditioned, they should be the same personality type—and they were.

The sixteen personality types easily divided into four different groups. Below is an overview of the four personality groups. I hope they offer some insight into the kind of awareness that is characteristic of each group. You can expect to identify these same characteristics in yourself and others when you practice the stretches that relate to each group. After looking briefly at descriptions of these four groups, we will look at descriptions of each personality type individually.

Note that the physical group focuses on the body and health, the spiritual group is aware of energy and life, the emotional group is conscious of looks and being, and the mental group is clear on knowing and understanding. You may have to step back to realize that your approach to life may be almost entirely through only one of these four

THE FOUR GENETIC PERSONALITY GROUPS				
	PHYSICAL	**SPIRITUAL**	**EMOTIONAL**	**THINKING**
Instinct	Anger/Love	Moral/Amoral	Excited/Anxious	Fearless/Fearful
Time reference	Present	Relative	Past	Future
Awareness	Awake/Asleep	Alive/Suffering	Conscious/Unconscious	Clear/Confused
Function	Active	Reactive	Retroactive	Proactive

windows. Notice the behavioral traits of others and recognize how yours may differ. How often do you stop and consider what motivates your behavior? Now perform the stretches associated with each group and notice how they affect your behavior.

The physical group of personality types (relates to the functioning of your lungs, thymus, skin, heart)

This group is concerned with the body. The four different types of stretches in this group make you aware of your instinct for love or for anger. You find yourself angry when a relationship is not going right, but otherwise you feel overwhelmingly and unconditionally loving. These stretches also make you aware of how to be present and active minded. You crave immediate results. These stretches also make you feel more awake and less anesthetized. It's as if you have just awakened from a great power nap and are incredibly alert and aware. And on your low end you find that your attention is all over the place. You are distracted and sleepy, and can't seem to find the wakefulness you need.

The spiritual group of personality types (relates to the functioning of your pericardium, appendix, large intestine, pancreas)

The four different types of stretches in this group make you aware of your moral instinct, what's right and what's wrong. You can't help but notice that not taking out the trash isn't fair to your roommate. You empathize easily with others and understand what makes them do what they do. These stretches also make you aware that time seems to be relative. Sometimes, when you are having fun, time moves very fast, but when you are doing something you don't enjoy, it seems to crawl. These stretches make you aware of feeling more energetically alive while removing your dullness and listlessness.

Emotional group of personality types (relates to the functioning of your liver, reproductive organs, bladder, small intestine)

The four types of stretches in this group can make you aware of what you are excited or anxious about. You are going to buy something you've been thinking about for a while and you're eager and delighted to wear it for the first time. But you haven't written the paper that's due tomorrow, even though you had a month to do it, and now the deadline hangs over your head like an axe and your anxiety is going through the roof. The stretches in this group can also make you aware of your past and how you need to process your experiences first before responding.

Thinking group of personality types (related to the functioning of your kidneys, brain, gallbladder, stomach)

The four types of stretches in this group can make you aware of becoming courageous and less afraid. You may have always been afraid of jumping off the fivemeter diving platform. Now you listen to your fear instinct, and you find yourself jumping even higher into the air so that your body can align itself to enter the water more easily. Your fear instinct shows you what to do so that you become fearless and proficient. These stretches also can make you look to the future and thus become more proactive in your decisions. You are working on things now that are connected to your career. You're always thinking of how your actions will affect your future. And these stretches can make you aware of just how clear or confused are your thoughts about something. You're on top of the world again, happy about what you know.

Once you begin to experience and identify the unique psychological instincts, time association, and awareness of each of the four personality groups, you will probably begin to perceive and target specific personality traits or behaviors that you want to grow or develop, as well as others that you'd like to leave behind. The stretching program presented in Chapters 9–13 can show you just how to do this. You'll also have the opportunity in Chapter 14 to measure your flexi-

bility for each of the sixteen genetic personality types and their traits in order to customize a stretching program that targets the specific traits that you would like to enhance.

Your new psychological understanding is intimately connected not just to your body but also to your breathing. There's some new information about your breathing that will help you to accept your psychological insights. Let's learn about new ways to breathe.

New Ways of Breathing

How to achieve simultaneous tension and relaxation

Everyone who has performed any type of strength training probably learned very early on that their body wanted them to inhale when they pushed or pulled the weight. It probably just felt natural to breathe in this way. You didn't have to think about it. It's what happens when you lift weight. When I began my own first attempts at stretching, I discovered that when stretching got especially intense, my breathing became very labored and difficult. I often found myself holding my breath. I reacted to my inability to breathe by deliberately attempting to control my inhalations and exhalations. And I tried to force myself to breathe in a number of self-conscious and intentional ways. Nothing worked. It took me a while to realize that any attempt to control my breathing was ultimately counterproductive.

I asked myself, "What *is* the best way to breathe?" I learned to pay close attention to the feeling that I was unable to breathe and then to wait patiently until my body showed me how to do it. This required unswerving trust in the involuntary instincts to breathe that were hardwired into my body. Many stretches disrupted and challenged my usual ability to breathe. This difficulty was obviously linked to habitual breathing patterns that surfaced when I stretched, exposing areas of tension in my body. Clearly I needed to change my old habits of breathing. I kept learning, switching my attention to the areas in my body where I was feeling the stretch and not on my breath and any attempts to manipulate it. By paying attention to the sensations I was experiencing while stretching, my mind was free to allow my breathing to regulate in whatever ways were necessary to stretch well.

Mechanics of Breathing

Your diaphragm is like a dome. Muscles contract and pull the dome downward as the ribs rise and expand on the inhale. When you exhale, the dome is released and stretches (probably the opposite of what you thought). If you view your diaphragm in this way, then when you're tight somewhere in your body, a part of this dome becomes warped—it is not allowed to move.

Some people habitually inhale more

and some people exhale more. Though you always need to exhale when performing the stretch, over time you will become more adept at balancing your inhales and exhales, and you will find that this "balancing act" begins to steady and poise your life in other more unconventional ways.

These are the simple mechanics of breathing when you stretch. But breathing involves much more than an inhalation of oxygen and exhalation of carbon dioxide. There is a life force—a regenerative energy—that flows through your physical body when you breathe. You will find as you continue to stretch that breathing determines your capacity to relax, enjoy, and learn while stretching.

Breathing Blueprints

Many of the new ways that I was learning to breathe were directly related to very positive experiences. For example, I discovered how to breathe the way someone who is loved breathes, instead of someone who is unloved. Or I breathed like someone who is positively affirmed and cared for, instead of someone who is neglected, put down, and denigrated. I learned that life-advancing events teach our bodies to breathe in really wonderful ways.

Any extra tension in your body directly prevents you from breathing fully. Removing tenseness in any area of the body, therefore, increases your ability to breathe. Remember: The tenseness that

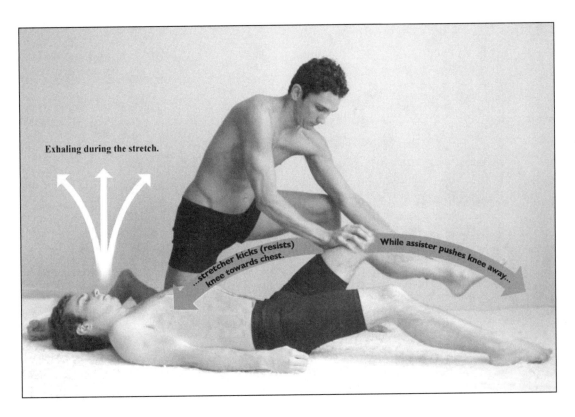

Exhaling during the stretch.

...stretcher kicks (resists) knee towards chest.

While assister pushes knee away...

you uncover while stretching will make you want to breathe in dramatic ways. Don't *make yourself* breathe smoothly, or deeply, or exclusively through your nose or mouth. Instead, find out how to breathe within each stretch—freely, naturally, and without conscious interference. I found that I couldn't know exactly how I was going to breathe until after it had happened. This is the secret behind really great breathing. As my skill level in stretching improved, it became easier for me to notice how my breathing was changing while I was stretching. After time, this constant effort at finding new ways to breathe became second nature.

A Few Key Points About Breathing

Exhale when stretching— Inhale when strengthening

Always exhale while moving and resisting during the stretch, and inhale when overcoming the resistance in strength training.

Keep your focus

Keep your attention on the sensations produced by what you are doing. Only by sticking your attention to sensations that are being produced by your stretch can your breathing change.

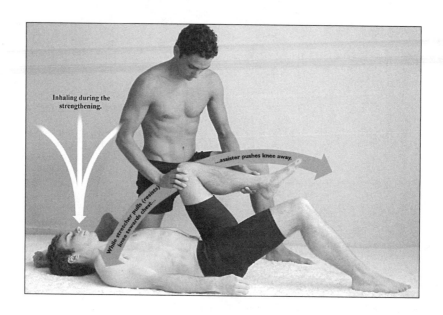

Inhaling during the strengthening.

While stretcher pulls (resists) knee towards chest...

...assister pushes knee away.

New breathing habits

Involuntary reflexes get you to breathe. Learning how to breathe differently for each activity builds upon this original instinctual reflex, giving you new ways of breathing that become second nature over time. Learn to attach to new ways of breathing and detach from old, unsuccessful ways of breathing.

The secret of breathing

You won't know precisely how you're going to breathe until after it has happened!

Tension and Relaxation

You cannot relax if you are not aware of your tenseness. As you become more and more aware of your internal tenseness, your breathing changes and causes you to relax. (Mentally dropping tenseness brings intenseness, not relaxation.)

The mechanics of breathing

Your diaphragm muscles stretch and rise on the exhalation and shorten and descend on the inhalation (probably the opposite of what you thought).

Effortlessness

To be as successful as you wish in different aspects of your life, you need to learn how to generate maximum tension with simultaneous relaxation.

Now let's spend a little more time examining these points in greater detail.

Effortlessness—Maximum Tension and Relaxation

When you stretch using maximum resistance, you know that you must generate incredible tension—maximum tension. But you must also be relaxed at the same time. This simultaneous tension and relaxation is present in many activities—sports, creativity, sex. It is especially true of stretching.

As you breathe naturally, you discover two very important phenomena. First, your tension redistributes itself over your entire body—collecting exactly where you need it and in just the right amounts—while it exits other places where it has been habitually held. Second, if you breathe naturally, your body simultaneously relaxes. This simultaneous tension-relaxation phenomenon is being effortless.

Although you perform more and more difficult stretches, at greater and greater levels of tension, if you breathe freely while you do them, you begin to feel more and more relaxed as you stretch. At times when I stretch, I find myself using surprising amounts of tension and relaxation concurrently. It is my breathing that is regulating this, not my thoughts. When you stretch, you need to generate maximum whole-body tension. Breathing can help you add relaxation to balance the tension and resistance you feel in your muscle. When your muscle reaches just the right amount of tension, a reflex fires and causes the muscle to lengthen further. After the fire reflex has occurred, the body experiences extraordinary levels of relaxation and release.

Good Looks, Good Moods, Good Energy, and Good Thinking!

What occurs inside you when you stretch and how you look on the outside are usually often quite the opposite of what you'd think. Surprisingly, the more tension you generate inside when stretching and breathing naturally, the more relaxed you will feel and look on the outside.

Just as my breathing affected my emotions and moods, it also affected my looks and my level of satisfaction with myself. The care I took to allow my body to breathe naturally absolutely determined my demeanor and physical attractiveness. As stretching matures you emotionally, you'll notice that you've become more honest, relaxed, and sexy—transporting you into deeply relaxed and intensely ecstatic states. Your bad moods will evaporate like fog, while your self-worth will break through like rays of sunshine.

Your new ways of breathing allow you to think more for yourself—to think outside the box. You literally begin to generate more of your own ideas that are grounded in your experiences.

Chapter 6

The Energy Flow Cycle

The natural order of things

WHEN MOST PEOPLE HEAR THAT resistance stretching involves stretching groups of muscles that are associated with energy meridians, they assume that I must have formally studied classical hatha yoga and traditional Chinese medicine (TCM) and then somehow combined these ancient systems of knowledge.

But I absolutely did not! I had few notions of classical hatha yoga or traditional Chinese medicine when I began to rediscover these ancient systems of knowledge. And it would have never dawned on me that they were somehow connected. When I first began to associate specific muscle groups with organ functions, I was baffled. I had no idea that certain muscles and organs might correlate to one another. But every time I stretched a particular muscle, I experienced an improvement in the same organ and not another organ. Other people had similar results without any prompting from me. And yes, the organ that was being affected by the stretch was located along the very muscles that energy meridians travel through the body to that organ.

After a while, to make things simple, I began to refer to various muscle groups by their associated organ in TCM. So, if I stretched the muscles on the outside of my lower body and torso, I'd say that I was stretching the Gallbladder muscles, which is what those muscles are associated with in TCM. Everyone who stretched in the stretching studio also began to refer to stretches by the muscle-meridian-organ associations of TCM. The vital energy or life force that I experienced moving through these energy meridians and organs was alien to my way of thinking at the time. But it opened me to a radical, albeit ancient, approach to healing and health.

When I later began reading about TCM, it contributed greatly to my understanding of how my body functions, the interrelationships of various parts of my body, and the definition and causes of various physical and psychological illnesses. The theories set forth in this book about muscle-organ correspondences, energy flow, and sequencing are all consistent. I've ventured beyond these theories and added a few new discoveries of my own.

Yin and Yang

In traditional Chinese medicine, each organ of the body has an energy line or muscle meridian pathway that traverses the body in the same way that channels move across Earth's surface. Meridians are not visible to the naked eye; they are located deep within skin tissue—pathways of energy that move up and down the body, distributing energy to and from one part of your body to another and from one organ to another.

Half of the meridians and organs are considered yin, and half are considered yang. The yin muscle meridians wrap from the front of your body around to the inside of your body, and the yang meridians wrap from the outside of your body around to the back of your body. There are eight yin and eight yang meridians. According to TCM, the energy that flows through these meridians is called chi. This vital flow and all-pervasive energy courses and eddies through every living thing, changing qualities according to the creative interplay between two mutually dependent, constantly changing forces called yin and yang. Yin is characterized by feminine principles—passive, expansive, cold, darkness, completion, submission, the moon. Yang is characterized by masculine principles—active, contractive, hot, brightness, hard, creation, dominance, the sun. Meridians affect every organ and physiological system, including immune, nervous, circulatory, endocrine, respiratory, skeletal, digestive, muscular, and lymphatic.

The Sixteen Self-Discovery Channels

I try not to limit my own thinking by what others before me have thought. I deeply appreciate and respect the ideas and innovations that have laid the groundwork for my own venturings. And, although I like to advance new theories, I am very careful not to lose the original premises when I make discoveries. I think of myself as starting where others leave off. In TCM, there are twelve regular meridians and several extraordinary channels. In my experience, however, I found that there were actually sixteen meridians with concomitant muscle groups and organs. I call these energy meridians the sixteen "self-discovery channels." Each of the sixteen channels has very specific muscle and organ associations. These four additional meridians, and the refined associations within each energy channel, are discussed further in Chapter 7.

How did I discover that there were sixteen and not twelve meridians? Well, I had uncovered stretches that affected all of the organs identified in TCM. But I had also identified four others that were not exactly known to TCM. What TCM refers to as "extraordinary channels" seemed to me to be a leaving-off place—a point of departure requiring further exploration. As I tried different stretches, I discovered four new energy pathways and corresponding organs. So I simply added these four to the twelve to arrive at the current roster of sixteen. I haven't found any others yet, but I'm open to the possibility!

The Natural Flow

After repeatedly experiencing an organ–muscle group association, something fun happened. After several months of stretching, I discovered that certain stretches just naturally felt good to do after some of the others. I came up with several different series of stretches, based on sequences of stretches that gave me a sense of joy. Each of these short flows of stretches seemed just naturally to connect one stretch to another, until four or more felt good together. No big deal, I thought, except I learned that the order in which I was practicing these little flows of stretches was very similar to the order of meridian energy flow through identical muscle groups in traditional Chinese medicine. According to TCM, energy passes from one meridian pathway into the next in a specific order. As energy flows sequentially from one meridian into the next, a flow series along the sixteen meridians is established. This energy flow in TCM is called the "energy cycle."

Many other fellow stretchers came up with similar flows that corresponded to TCM. I then connected all the small flows together so that all the muscles of the body could be stretched in a single routine. I called this an "energy series." An energy series is composed of sixteen different types of stretches practiced in a very specific order; each stretch refers to an organ and its energy meridian in TCM.

I'd like to note, however, that just because I or anyone else likes to progress through stretches in a particular order, this absolutely does not mean that you will or should do your stretches in that order. I present four energy series in this book, beginner, intermediate, assisted, and advanced. Please feel free to do your stretches in whatever sequencing you like best. A worksheet in Chapter 14 allows you to put together your own sequence. There are many personal reasons why you might need to follow a different sequence, as you will discover as you read this book. I'm 100 percent behind self-discovery and doing what feels right.

The Energy Flow Series

My preferred order of stretches is illustrated in the diagram above right. Flows are usually thought of as a circle, so I have placed the flow order of stretches around this circle with their organ concomitance. You will notice that we start with the superficial muscles and move inward toward the deeper muscles.

I prefer to show the energy flow on a ladder or trellis shape shown at right (it is actually the trellis opening to my organic garden). Next to each numbered stretch in the series is the energy meridian or organ that is affected by that stretch. For example: #1 (GB) is the first stretch, and the muscles you are stretching are identical to the muscles along the gallbladder energy meridian

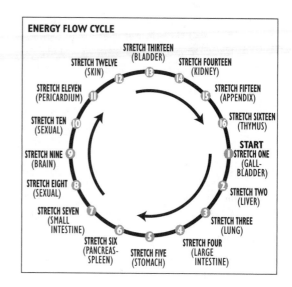

in TCM. The numbers also correspond to the numbered stretches in the energy stretch series offered a little later in this book. Here's the rose garden trellis diagram:

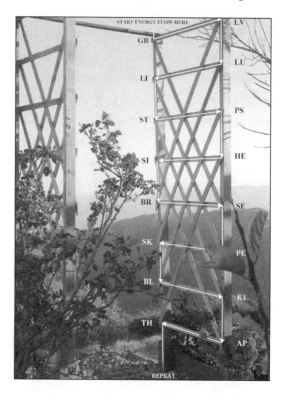

(Note that the order begins with two leg muscle groups, then two arm muscle groups, and then repeats.)

The Interrelationships Among Meridians and Muscles

There are sixteen meridian-muscle groups—eight in your lower body and eight in your upper body. The simple diagram on page 54, representing the energy series, also explains very important interrelationships among those meridian-muscle groups. Let's delve a little deeper.

In the rose trellis diagram, the horizontal pairs are balancing organs in TCM, but they are also balancing muscle groups. In Western anatomy, balancing muscle groups are called agonists and antagonists. For example, the stomach (ST) meridian-muscle group is located on the front side of your body, and its balancing muscle group is the pancreas-spleen (PS) meridian-muscle group, which is exactly opposite, on the back inside of your body. When one of these groups stretches, the other must shorten and reverse.

This balancing relationship is important for many reasons, but in particular it means that if you cannot get a good stretch in one group it is probably because its balancing muscle group can't shorten enough to get you into a position to stretch. So knowing about balancing relationships gives

you the data to fix what may be faltering and get it to work.

The diagram also houses other secrets about the interrelationships of muscles, organs, and personalities. For example, the numbered stretches directly above and below each other are actually the exact muscle groups above and below in your body. One is in your arms and one is in your legs. For example, directly above the stomach group is the large intestine group. The lower-body muscles in the ST group correspond to the upper-body muscles in the LI group. So when you want to stretch the same muscles above and below, you can use the trellis to tell you which muscles these are. We call these "completing" meridian-muscle groups.

The Body . . . Universe in Microcosm

Your body in traditional Chinese medicine is understood as both internally stable and dynamic. Its flexibility allows it to adapt to constant changes and fluctuations in both the internal and external environment. In this holistic view, an organic connection exists among organs, their related tissues, and your life.

This is a systems view of the body. The body is seen as an elegantly organized, self-regulating universe—a complex system of interdependent interactions among many working parts. Energy meridians follow this systems view. They bring vitality and balance, adjust the body's metabolism, remove blockages, and impact cellular change. Meridian energies are designed to help the body self-heal and to restore homeostasis and harmony. Contemporary life, with its attendant stresses, toxins, and depletions, constantly threatens these energies and can result in ill health. Much faith, then, is vested in the ability to heal oneself through a balancing of these energies, as well as a balancing of one's inner and outer lives.

Uncanny Connections

The fascinating connection among sixteen muscle groups, sixteen meridians, and sixteen personality types is just one example of concomitance. Once you've experienced that stretching a certain muscle group creates an improvement, not just in your physical flexibility but also in the physiological functioning of a particular organ, you can then begin to make other connections between muscle groups and other aspects of yourself and your life.

As surprising as it may have been to you that your digestive or immunological system could be upgraded by stretching specific muscles, you can also look for other changes to occur. You'll probably discover that past physical traumas or injuries can be removed and replaced with a better ability to move than you had before, while at the same time, you will notice distinct changes in your moods and affect. It's not much of a leap to understand that your body can re-

flect past events, emotions (both old and new), and things that are happening in your life in the here and now.

So you've learned that the sixteen stretches correspond to a meridian-muscle group. This association between types of stretches and their ability to access and produce specific benefits is called a concomitance. When one thing is inseparably connected or associated to another thing, there is said to be a concomitance between those two things. As you've now learned, there is a direct correspondence between muscle groups and meridian pathways and organs. But there are additional benefits that are known to be concomitant with each of the sixteen types of stretches. These benefits—collected from thousands of people's experiences—can be grouped into categories of concomitance.

For example, each of the sixteen types of stretches can improve the physiological functioning of a particular organ, repair a specific type of tissue, and bring forth specific personality traits. Each of the sixteen can also allow you to experience a specific way of breathing. Bear in mind that a concomitant relationship between two things explicitly demands that one thing always bring with it the other . . . they have an inseparable relationship.

Basic Concomitance

The theory of concomitance implies that when you stretch certain groups of muscles along an organ-energy meridian, the organ is affected positively. But concomitance is a two-way street. The effects go both ways. This means that if you affect the health of an organ through the use of dietary supplements, then the muscle group associated with that organ will also become healthier and more flexible. Or if you develop a specific high personality trait, let's say being more empathic, this mental change can result in an upgrade in your pancreas, and the associated muscle group will become healthier and more flexible. Or if you affect the health of a type of tissue in your body by stretching, then it can affect your ability to develop particular high personality traits.

There are many parallels, some more apparent than others. It is obvious to everyone that physical exercise improves the physical body, but for many it is a stretch of the imagination to believe that physical exercise can provide direct improvements in what happens to you in your life, or that it can affect your emotional development or change you psychologically—or change the world. So stretches for specific muscle groups, concomitant organs, and personality traits all function in a mutually interdependent relationship.

The Four Aspects of Stretching

The largest and most obvious truth about stretching is that if you are truly flexible,

then you are flexible not just physically but also spiritually, emotionally, and mentally. Being flexible in all four ways is not difficult and is not a mystery. The position of each stretch corresponds to your body's physical health and the options that you have in your life. The resistance of the stretch corresponds to your spiritual development. The breathing of the stretch corresponds to the level of satisfaction you have in your desires and in your emotional maturity. And the mental part of the stretch corresponds to your psychological fitness and character development. This basic concomitance between the four parts of stretching and the four parts of yourself (body, spirit, emotion, and breathing) is pictured below.

You are physically flexible when you are agile, supple, and childlike in your movements. You are spiritually flexible when you are open-minded, empathetic, appreciative, and yielding. You are emotionally flexible when you are mature, sexy, honest, and passionate. And you are men-

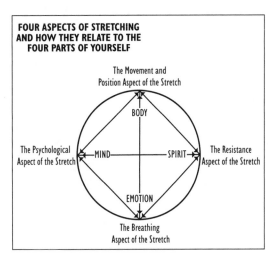

FOUR ASPECTS OF STRETCHING AND HOW THEY RELATE TO THE FOUR PARTS OF YOURSELF

The Movement and Position Aspect of the Stretch

BODY

The Psychological Aspect of the Stretch — MIND — SPIRIT — The Resistance Aspect of the Stretch

EMOTION

The Breathing Aspect of the Stretch

tally flexible when you are sober, decisive, masterful, and understanding.

For example, if you stretch and improve the flexibility of muscles on the back of your shoulder, your arm will have greater flexibility and strength—thus affecting you physically. But you'll also experience an improvement in the assimilation of your food, because the health of your small intestine has improved—thus achieving a physiological improvement. And you'll become more creative and less depressed—a mental or psychological improvement. And you'll experience yourself being more positively affirming—experiencing a spiritual affect. Or you could take a specific herb for your small intestine, and not only would you derive improvements in your physiological health, but your arm would become more flexible and strong, and you would become more creative and self-affirming.

Actively working on any one of the four aspects of yourself—physical, spiritual, emotional, and mental—brings concurrent improvements in the other three aspects and is concomitant with one of the sixteen different parts of yourself. This is the principle of concomitance. The only way you can have all four dimensions of flexibility is by developing all four aspects for each of the sixteen stretches. Don't focus only on the physical part! While this book introduces new stretching techniques and stretches that allow you to become more physically flexible than you ever thought possible, the extraordinary uniqueness of resistance stretching—and this book—is that these stretches provide the opportunity to develop spiritually, emotionally, and psychologically as well.

Connected but Not the Same

Before we consider all the different connections between the four parts, we need to be clear about what concomitance does not mean. When you develop your body in a specific way, you can expect a change in your personality. But not totally! You will still need to work directly on your personality in other ways in order to fully develop that part of you. Or you could develop yourself spiritually and your body would change, but you would still have to work on your body directly before you could expect the kind of physical changes you desire. The connection alone is not sufficient to bring about total change to the other.

It is extremely important to understand that a connection between two things does not make the two things the same. The

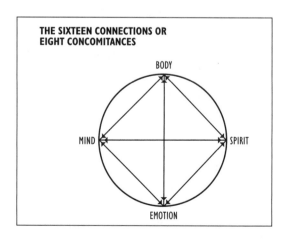

THE SIXTEEN CONNECTIONS OR EIGHT CONCOMITANCES

BODY

MIND

SPIRIT

EMOTION

connection allows both parts to be separate entities and still be one through the connection and thus affect one another. Relationships can be seen as two individuals that are also one! The connection indicates that both parts need to be worked on separately as well as through the connection.

The Sixteen Connections

Everyone knows that becoming more physically fit improves your physiological health. This is a *body-body connection*. Likewise, your life affects your energy (a *spirit-spirit connection*), your attachments affect your satisfaction (an *emotion-emotion connection*), and your clarity affects your mental mastery (a *mind-mind connection*). And most people have heard of the *mind-body connection* that, by affecting the way they think, improves their body's health. Likewise there is also a *body-mind connection*, in which, if you take tension out of a specific area in your body, your mind will become clear and unblocked in a particular way as well. But that's not the whole story.

Everyone has emotions and spiritual parts of themselves, and these parts must also connect with your body and your mind. There are sixteen permutations between one part of yourself and all the others. So in addition to the connections we just mentioned, there is also a *body-spirit and spirit-body connection*, a *body-emotion and emotion-body* connection, a *spirit-emotion and emotion-spirit* connection, *a spirit-mind and mind-spirit* connection, and a *mind-emotion* and *emotion-mind* connection—in total sixteen kinds of connections!

Becoming more flexible in different types of stretches essentially teaches you significantly different and remarkable ways of being connected to everything. Let's now see how all these connections form what I call the magic sixteen.

Chapter 7

The Magic Sixteen

Sixteen different stretches, sixteen muscle groups,
sixteen energy meridians, and sixteen personalities

WHEN I FIRST BEGAN STRETCHING, I didn't have the slightest idea how many types of stretches there might be. I was simply trying to create specific stretches for various areas of my body that required repair. I found sixteen types of stretches for the whole body. But as I mentioned in the first chapter, stretches mysteriously began naturally to define themselves around specific muscle groups and, within a short while, I had fourteen different types of stretches for the fourteen different muscle groups. It took six more years before the final two groups were added for a total of sixteen different groups of muscles—eight muscle groups in the legs and eight muscle groups in the arms. So the stretches and their corresponding muscle groups matched up.

While developing these stretches, I was simultaneously experiencing the improvement of specific organ functions—from my heart to my intestines to my brain. That these physiological functions were being affected was surprising enough, but it was the realization that specific stretches caused particular and predictable physiological functions to change and reverse themselves that was truly mind-boggling. When other people began to experience these same muscle-organ concomitances, the idea that muscles and organs were connected became more and more difficult to resist. Then, a close friend told me that the same exact correlation between these sixteen specific muscle groups and the sixteen meridians and their organ associations that I was experiencing was already defined in the theories of traditional Chinese medicine. So these sixteen meridian pathways literally traversed the sixteen different muscle groups that I had developed stretches for.

Likewise, I had noticed that specific stretches were affecting me in very particular ways psychologically, and that other people who performed these stretches were also experiencing the same distinct changes in affect, behavior, and speech. Stretches had the capacity to lift a person out of negative states and transport him or her back into opposite high personality traits. And of course, these psychological traits—particular to different types of stretches—also totaled sixteen! Shortly, these experiences evolved into my own theory of sixteen genetic personality types—the sixteen geniuses. The stretches, the muscle groups, the energy meridians, and the personality types all matched up!

So I had unexpectedly uncovered sixteen types of stretches, sixteen muscle-meridian groups, and sixteen personality types. And the stretches, the muscle groups, the energy meridians, and the personality types all matched up! That's why we call the stretches "the magic sixteen." These sixteen body stretches introduced me to a new and mind-expanding (not to mention spirit- and emotion-expanding!) dimension. And they have ushered in countless occurrences of spontaneous healing and positive life transformations for everyone who has become involved.

Sixteen—A Magic Number

So there are sixteen different stretches, sixteen muscle groups, sixteen meridian pathways, and sixteen genetic personality types:

- There are sixteen different stretches—eight stretches for your legs and eight stretches for your arms (doing all sixteen stretches in a particular order is an Energy Series).
- There are sixteen muscle groups—eight different muscle groups in your lower body and eight different muscle groups in your upper body (these are the muscle-meridian groups).
- There are also sixteen meridian pathways in TCM—eight traversing through the muscles in your lower body and eight traversing through the muscles in your upper body (these are the sixteen self-discovery channels).
- And, finally, there are sixteen genetic personality types (GPT)—four physical types, four spiritual types, four emotional types, and four mental types (the sixteen geniuses).

Yes, each of the sixteen different types of stretches can be used to increase the flexibility (or strength) of one muscle group that corresponds exactly to one meridian, and that corresponds to exactly one type of genius. Everything matches up—all sixteen stretches, sixteen muscle groups, sixteen meridians, and sixteen personality types pair up with each other exactly.

The Sixteen Different Types of Stretches

The sixteen different types of stretches are described in Part III. There you will find beginner, intermediate, assisted, and advanced sets of sixteen stretches in each series.

The Sixteen Muscle-Meridian Groups

There are hundreds of muscles in your body. Is there a way that they are naturally organized that makes it easy to understand them? Yes. Different stretches involve not just a single muscle but groups of muscles. There are only sixteen different groups of muscles in you body, eight in your upper body and eight in your lower body.

Here's an easy way to visualize them. When you look at your body from above as a circle, there are eight groups of muscles in both your lower and upper body. There are muscles on the front (anterior) and back (posterior), muscles on the inside (medial)

and outside (lateral), and on the four angles. Here's what it looks like:

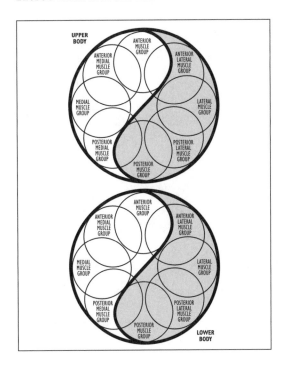

If you think of your legs and arms schematically as circles and view them from above, then there are eight muscle-meridian groups in your lower body and eight muscle-meridian groups in your upper body. Note that each group consists of its own specific muscles spanning a 45-degree arc about this circle and also shares a few muscles with its neighboring group.

These same muscle groups can be viewed also as TCM meridian-organ pathways. So in your lower body, your front muscle group is called the sexual meridian muscle group, your back muscle group is called the brain meridian muscle group, etc. Here are the same sixteen muscle groups as described in Eastern medicine.

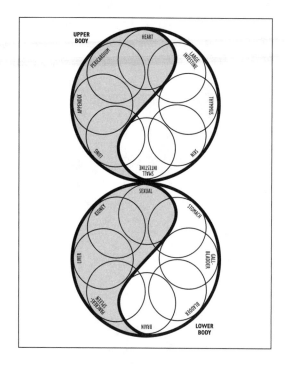

The Sixteen Meridian Pathways of Traditional Chinese Medicine

Here are the actual TCM energy meridians. Note that each meridian is named by the organ that is associated with it. There are, of course, sixteen!

The Sixteen Genetic Personality Types— the Sixteen Geniuses

As you know, there are four personality groups—physical, spiritual, emotional, and thinking—and four types within each group,

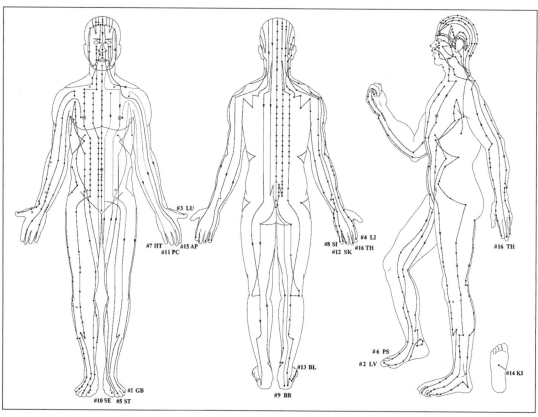

totalling sixteen personality types. Each personality type has its own exceptional high qualities. These qualities are so prevalent in their daily actions that I have come to see them as genius traits, so I call the sixteen personality types the sixteen geniuses. Here are each personality type's best genius qualities.

Physical types

Leader: the genius of truthfulness and power (lungs)

Healer: the genius of healing and forgiveness (thymus)

Challenger: the genius of athleticism and community (skin)

Lover: the genius of unconditional love and action (heart)

Spiritual types

Judge: the genius of judiciousness and openness (pericardium)

Individualist: the genius of change and transformation (appendix)

Perfectionist: the genius of perfection and completion (large intestine)

Peacemaker: the genius of peacefulness and communication (pancreas-spleen)

Emotional types

Helper: the genius of freedom and giving (liver)

God(dess): the genius of sexuality and will (sexual)

Performer: the genius of honesty and hopefulness (bladder)

Artist: the genius of creativity and affirmations (small intestine)

Thinking types

Philosopher: the genius of understanding and humor (kidneys)

Master: the genius of responsibility and problem solving (brain)

Decision maker: the genius of decision making and devotion (gallbladder)

Soberer: the genius of sobriety and self-expression (stomach)

A Magic Correspondence

How all sixteen types of stretches, sixteen muscle groups, sixteen meridians, and sixteen personality types–geniuses correspond exactly is the magic behind resistance stretching. All the pieces of the puzzle form the big picture.

In this book, everything relates to the number of the stretches! For example, every energy series of stretches is numbered from 1 to 16. The flex tests, one for each of the four dimensions of yourself—physical, spiritual, emotional, and mental—all have sixteen questions corresponding exactly to the sixteen stretch numbers. Those questionnaires will allow you to begin to discover many things about yourself and others that you have probably always wondered about. You will begin to identify many different traits about yourself and other people.

All the recommended stretches for prevention and treatment of injuries, to

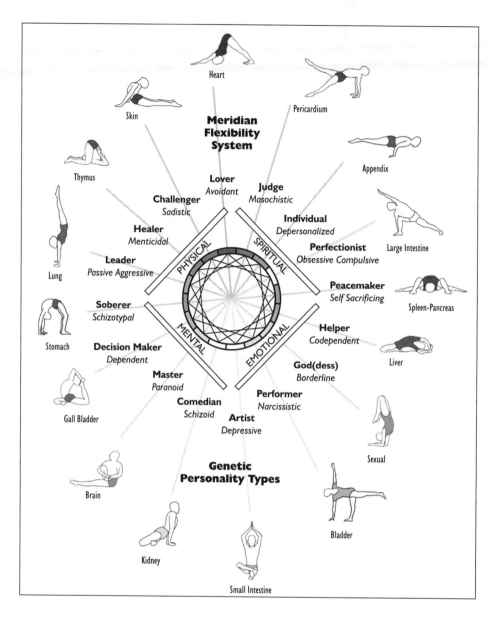

Heart

Pericardium

Skin

Meridian Flexibility System

Appendix

Thymus

Lover *Avoidant* **Judge** *Masochistic*

Challenger *Sadistic* **Individual** *Depersonalized*

Healer *Menticidal* **Perfectionist** *Obsessive Compulsive* Large Intestine

Leader *Passive Aggressive*

PHYSICAL SPIRITUAL

Lung

Peacemaker *Self Sacrificing* Spleen-Pancreas

Soberer *Schizotypal*

MENTAL EMOTIONAL

Helper *Codependent*

Stomach

Decision Maker *Dependent* Liver

God(dess) *Borderline*

Master *Paranoid*

Performer *Narcissistic*

Gall Bladder

Comedian *Schizoid*

Artist *Depressive*

Sexual

Brain

Genetic Personality Types

Bladder

Kidney

Small Intestine

promote health and prevent illness, to detox, and to increase your sexual satisfaction are referred to by the sixteen numbered stretches.

When you realize that stretching certain muscles can actually impact nonphysical areas in your life, you can begin to tailor your stretching to affect the issues or goals that are important to you. You will identify which of the four worldviews you need to know more about in order to be more balanced. You will specify what within each of those groups you need to work on specifically. Then, stretch back and watch how magical life becomes!

Chapter 8

Natural Stretching Movements and Using Resistance to Stretch

Discovering stretch moves

STRETCHES ARE DISCOVERED THROUGH personal experimentation and are only later analyzed and their benefits proved by scientific methods. Stretches are like secret formulas, trademark products that are viewed as sacred by those who create them. The most obvious and simplest stretches have been created through persistent and intense efforts by impassioned individuals—that's the genius sneaking through again. These simple stretches have become the most common everyday stretch movements that today we all take for granted. Classic stretch movements are much more difficult to create than you might imagine. So let's try to find out how to create them.

Your body begins by showing you how to stretch, and then your spirit, breathing, and mind want to join in. Discovering stretches is a creative process—it feels as if you pull the ideas out of thin air. It is an inspired endeavor that is so fluid and seemingly unconscious that you find yourself hoping that you can remember what you just did so you can repeat it the next time! That's why it's a great idea to have a friend close by to help you remember what you've created.

What you want to know about stretching will often be taught to you by others, as you connect what's known to them to what's inside you. But a lot of the time you will teach yourself. Quite quickly it will become obvious to you that no one could scientifically "think up" stretches, for even the simplest stretches incorporate an enormous number of mind-boggling bone interrelationships. For example, your thigh can move in twenty-seven different ways, but so can your lower leg, and your ankle and foot. That creates $27 \times 27 \times 27 =$ approximately 30,000 possible movements for just one of your legs. Add your other leg and two arms, and you're in the trillions of possible movements. So it's easy to see that letting your body show you how to stretch is a much more preferred method of designing stretches. (Later, if you become interested in analyzing and proving the scientific effectiveness of the stretch and strengthening exercises in this book, you can read about the scientific analysis of those exercises on our Web page.)

As you experiment, you'll discover stretches that feel natural and inborn, as if they've been waiting for you to liberate them. You can't wait to see what your body comes up with next!

The Starting Point

In weight training, you start in a position where you elongate the muscle you want to build, and then contract and shorten the muscle against additional resistance. In resistance stretching, the starting position is the opposite of weight training. You start at a point where the muscles you want to stretch are as short as possible, and then you contract and resist while those muscles are lengthened.

Thus, the only difference between weight training and flexibility training is that the starting positions and movements are opposite. But in both cases, you need to contract the muscles you're working on against added resistance. It's that simple when you think about it.

Seven Different Types of Movements for Stretching

There are different ways to approach stretching, and each offers specific benefits. Here's an explanation of seven forms of stretching and their advantages. Try them all.

I. Reposing

Have you ever watched animals lying around—or hanging around—in unusual positions and wondered why they do what they do? It's been my experience that different poses affect the health of my organs and my physiological and psychological well-being in very specific ways. So when a dog lies on her back, exposing her belly to the sun, I've found that I do that too when-

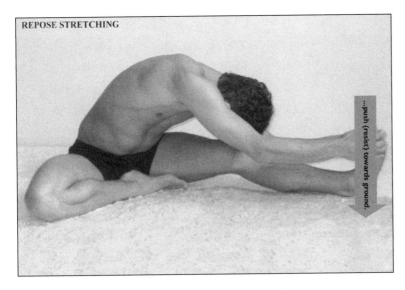

REPOSE STRETCHING

...push (resist) towards ground.

stretching is constantly contracting, but this contraction is involuntary and perhaps unconscious to most people. The longer you stay in a pose, the greater the tension level in those muscles you are stretching becomes. Though repose stretches may appear to be relaxing, inside they are generating enormous tension involuntarily to stretch specific muscles.

ever I want to calm my stomach. Perhaps the dog calms herself this way too! A cat stretches his hind legs behind him and rests his head on his front paws. Well, I do this too—to destress myself and turn on my external immune system. Birds often stand very still before arching or flexing their necks to shake off the kinks, just the way people do when they're uptight and need to deescalate and settle into themselves better.

Just like animals, we look for natural repose positions that make us feel better, calmer, or safer. If specific muscles need recovery, or specific organs need rejuvenating, or we need to regroup psychologically, it is important that we find ways to help ourselves. We need to learn to curl and coil into repose positions that rejuvenate the parts of ourselves that are sore or stressed. These are healing positions that humans, just like animals, also need to learn and enjoy. But don't forget that in these apparently passive positions, any muscle you are

Repose stretching is used primarily for recovery and recharging yourself after feeling depleted or ill. It is also a great way to regroup and relax during times of anxiety or distress.

2. Natural dynamic movements

Every time you run, jump, kick, throw, or just fool around, your muscles are being passively strengthened and stretched. So all movement stretches you passively. Some people call this dynamic stretching because you are moving. Most sports move you in only so many different ways, get into only so many different kinds of positions, so you need to do different sports to stretch and strengthen every part of you.

3. Isometric stretching

When you are in a static position and voluntarily pushing (resisting) against the floor, wall, or yourself, you are resisting. This in-

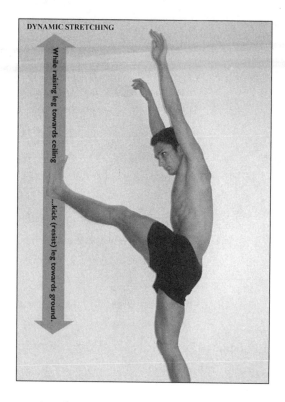

DYNAMIC STRETCHING

While raising leg towards ceiling

...kick (resist) leg towards ground.

Many end positions are locked and you cannot move, so isometric resistance is the only way to get a great active stretch. As a matter of fact, in most yoga postures you cannot move and thus need to resist in order to generate a stretch.

4. Resistance stretching

Birds elaborately spread and resistance-stretch their wings before they fly. Cats and dogs regularly stretch with resistance before they get up to run after a nap. And we humans stretch and resist with our arms and legs before we get out of bed in the morning.

Everyone knows that you use additional weight (resistance) when you strength-train to increase gains. And as you discovered earlier, the key to flexibility is stretching and also using resistance—just like a cat. As you move in and out of a particular stretch, you learn

tentional resistance results in the muscles stretching, and though it looks like nothing is moving from outside yourself, your bones are subtly changing their relationships.

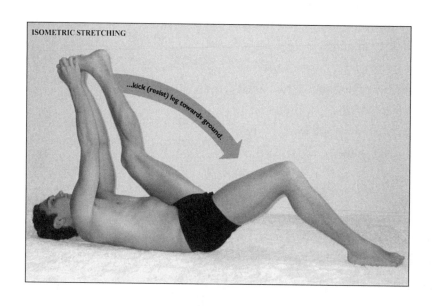

ISOMETRIC STRETCHING

...kick (resist) leg towards ground

how to use resistance to produce the stretch by pushing against the floor, a wall, or yourself. All of the sixty-four stretches offered in this book incorporate resistance while you stretch. Move and resist = stretching . . . repeat . . . focus on a different muscle group . . . move and resist = stretching . . . repeat . . .

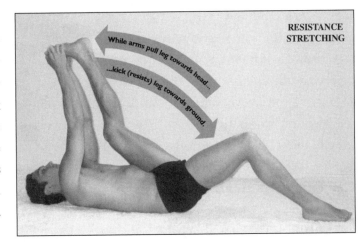

RESISTANCE STRETCHING

While arms pull leg towards head..

...kick (resists) leg towards ground

Attempting and practicing different stretches repetitively—using resistance, of course—facilitates final mastery of a stretch and can be used to target or troubleshoot specific inflexibilities.

5. Stretch flows

Sixteen kinds of stretches are included in each stretch routine offered in this book (what I call the energy flow series). Instead of practicing a particular movement, resisting to produce the stretch, and then simply repeating it a number of times, the energy flow series allows you to move from one kind of stretch into another, then another, until you complete all sixteen stretches covering your whole body. Your muscles are passively strengthened and stretched when you move. For example, when you kick your leg into the air in front of you, the muscles on the front of your thigh are being passively strengthened while the muscles on the back of your thigh are being passively

stretched. All free movement passively strengthens and stretches you.

Flows are particularly great for improving respiration and coordination, and they allow you to cover all the sixteen muscle groups. Your physical power increases from practicing stretching flows.

6. Stretching for psychological insight

When you spend many minutes or even hours practicing the same stretch, you enter into the personality type associated with the specific muscles you are stretching. Observing what you think, how your perception of things changes, and what personality traits come to the foreground occurs initially only by remaining in a stretch position for a long time. After a while, you will be able to identify psychological changes for each stretch.

As you begin to experience the unique nature of the personality type associated with a specific stretch, you will be broadened and educated psychologically in new and unexpected ways. Groups of people performing the same type of stretch for more than a half hour speak about how they experience the unique nature of the personality type associated with that stretch. They use identical words to describe how that stretch allows them to perceive the world outside themselves in a distinctly different way. Each of these experiences not only expands them personally but also creates the potential for more global change—transforming how they interact and engage with one another personally and at the level of community. (See Chapter 14 for examples of the psychological impacts of stretching.)

7. Being assisted or using equipment

We all want to be able to do things for ourselves, and the first three energy series provide very effective stretches that you can do by yourself. But you can no more do stretching by yourself than you can cut your own hair, fix your car, fix your teeth, or learn most things. Everything you do usually requires help from others, and stretching is no exception.

When other people assist you in stretches, you have the opportunity to generate much greater resistance, thus deriving far greater increases in flexibility than you could ever accomplish by yourself. As you push or pull against someone else, your muscles resist maximally. Wow! The results are dramatic increases in flexibility and strength.

Stop Struggling! Get into Great Positions

What is the secret to getting into great stretch positions and movements? In every stretch, some muscles shorten and pull you into the stretch while other muscles lengthen and stretch. It is commonly understood that when you are inflexible, you have a limited range of motion because the muscles you are stretching are tight. But what is not known is that often the muscles that need to contract and shorten to pull you into a stretch are unable to shorten enough to get you into a great position to stretch. Yes, it's not just that the muscles that you are trying to stretch are too tight, but other muscles can't contract enough ever to get you into a position that will give you the stretch you want. Why?

Every muscle needs to be able to stretch before it can shorten. Only if a muscle is sufficiently flexible is it capable of contracting and shortening enough. So if your muscle is maximally flexible, then you can contract and shorten it to get a great stretch where you want. Otherwise your stretch is limited. This is a very important principle usually unknown to and overlooked by everyone who stretches.

Maximum Resistance

Resistance stretching

Once you're moving in the stretch, your body naturally resists any elongation and attempts to move in the opposite direction you are pulling it. It always tries to return to the starting position. Consider the hamstring stretch you tried earlier. As you lay on your back and lifted your lower leg toward your head to stretch your hamstrings, did you notice that your lower leg resisted this elongation and pulled back down to your glutes? Your hamstrings lengthen but contract automatically . . . involuntarily. This involuntary contraction is resistance.

As you move into a stretch, your muscles lengthen—but they also contract. As the stretched muscles contract, tension develops and, at a certain point, a reflex fires and tells the muscles to elongate further. Now you're stretching! That's how it happens. It's that simple.

Resistance is not only natural but also necessary for any muscle to stretch. Tension and resistance must occur, because this is what causes the muscle to stretch. Your body naturally produces tension when it does this resistance thing. When you increase the resistance by intentionally fighting the elongation by resisting in the opposite direction of the stretch, the muscle actually produces double the tension and resistance that it does in weight training the same muscle, and the result is a dramatic increase in flexibility.

How to get a stretch without pain

There are illusions about flexibility that may be hard to see through at first. Some-one who can do full splits is generally assumed to be more flexible than someone who has a difficult time touching his or her toes. But surprisingly, this is not necessarily true. What I am about to say is not how flexibility is traditionally defined or understood.

Muscles generate twice the tension when stretching than when weight training. This means you have to use twice the force to stretch a muscle as to strengthen it. That's right. If you can lift fifty pounds, it takes 100 pounds to stretch the same muscle. This explains why few people become more flexible simply by elongating their muscles in traditional stretching—no increases in their flexibility occur, because they do not know to contract muscles while elongating them, and twice the force that a muscle could lift is not used to stretch it.

I have discovered that a muscle is truly flexible only when it is being lengthened and can simultaneously maximally resist. This ability to maximally resist throughout a certain range defines true functional ranges of movement where substitution is not occurring. Anytime you get yourself into a range of motion where you cannot maximally resist, you are overstretching and moving weirdly somewhere else. Therefore, someone who has little apparent range of motion but is able to maximally resist during that range is more flexible than a person with an overstretched range of motion.

This explains the apparent contradiction that sometimes someone who seems

When lengthening a muscle to test its flexibility, at the point where the muscle can no longer maintain a maximal contraction is its true flexibility range.

True flexibility occurs only when a muscle can contract maximally throughout its entire stretch length.

tighter performs better in sports than someone who seems looser. This is because he is actually more flexible than the apparently looser person. That looser person cannot maximally contract the muscles that seem to be showing impressive ranges of motion. He is also much more prone to injury. (Don't confuse this example with someone who is truly overly stiff and who constantly injures himself because of his inflexibility, or the truly very flexible person who moves with the grace of God.)

Discover this for yourself. Try again the hamstring stretch that you did to discover resistance stretching. Lie on your back, bring one knee to your chest, bend your lower leg, and grab your foot with both hands. Contract your hamstring and resist as your hands pull your heel toward your head. Now repeat the stretch, only now maximally resist the whole time. The point at which while pulling your heel toward your head you can no longer continue to resist maximally is the true flexibility range of your hamstrings. This length or flexibility range is obviously much less than if you resist only moderately and especially if you don't resist at all. When you maximally resist and pull your heel toward your head, you can measure the true flexibility of your hamstrings.

Here's another example. Someone who appears to have much less range of motion than someone else might very possibly be more flexible spiritually, emotionally, or psychologically than the physically flexible person who contorts her body to an extreme degree. Only when you have proper position, enough resistance, and appropriate ways of breathing, and can identify the psychological effects do you become

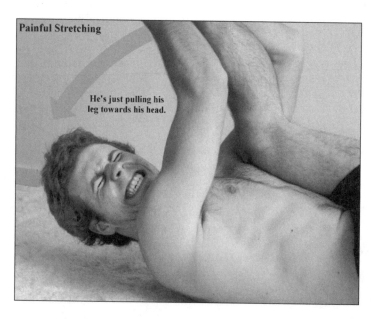

Painful Stretching

He's just pulling his leg towards his head.

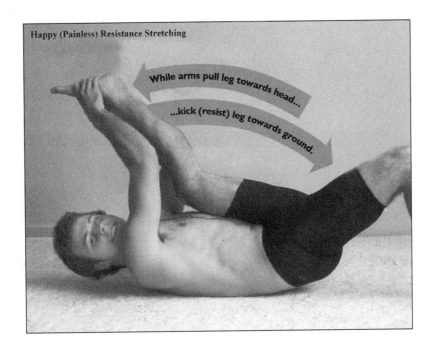

Happy (Painless) Resistance Stretching

While arms pull leg towards head...

...kick (resist) leg towards ground.

truly flexible in all ways in that particular stretch. Of course, being flexible in one stretch does not mean you are flexible in all stretches. Every person and every stretch is different.

Body tensions are usually the result of habitual actions and patterns of behavior that we have established in response to past trauma, current stresses, and even to lifestyle (the way we choose to live). As we watch these tensions reveal themselves, we begin to notice dramatic changes in respiration.

The Critical Difference

Try not to interfere with this natural resistance reaction. Your body has begun to move to a different drumbeat. It is one of the truly transformative aspects of this new type of stretching. And it brings the body to new levels of endurance, resiliency, and power.

Often I have heard stretchers observe how resistance stretching seems to remove the physical "inessentials" from their bodies. After stretching the arms of one of my athletes one day, he exclaimed, "I feel as if there's less junk in this arm. I could do *anything* with this arm now. I could learn to paint a picture, conduct a symphony, play the piano . . ."

One of the misconceptions I constantly confront about resistance stretching is the perception that it doesn't give the body the workout it requires for increasing strength, power, and stamina. However, my current work with Olympic athletes demonstrates that quite the opposite is true. Resistance stretching oftentimes exceeds all other forms of exercise in intensity and use of force.

Eli Fairfield, Olympic volleyball player, had this to say about resistance stretching: "I never did stretching before because, quite simply, it didn't work, so I was resistant to try other forms of stretching. The moment I tried resistance stretching, I got immediate changes in my flexibility. These changes translated into immediate increases in my speed and power when playing volleyball. I stretch every day now, and every athlete that sees me stretch asks me to teach them."

The Principle of Resistance

You must contract the muscle you are lengthening while stretching it. You begin to stretch by first placing your body in a position where you maximally shorten the muscle you are going to stretch. Then you contract the muscle and move in such a way as to lengthen the muscle. Both the contraction and the lengthening must occur simultaneously when stretching. Lengthening a muscle without contracting it at the same time overstretches the muscle and dramatically increases your risk of injury. Remember, it takes twice the tension to stretch a muscle as it does to strengthen it.

> Stretching is simultaneously resisting the lengthening of the muscle by contracting as the muscle is lengthened.

The Key Is Leverage

Once you know to use resistance when stretching, it becomes very obvious to you that you need good leverage. You have to be in a position where you can overcome the resistance that you are using while stretching. In order to have greater leverage, you might need to position yourself against a wall, or place yourself in a particular orientation to gravity.

The exact direction you move toward to produce the greatest stretch feels like the path of greatest resistance. Slightly altering the angle of your movement allows you to find exactly the best path to move through so that you feel you are pulling the tension right out of that part of your body. Let's consider an example or two about getting yourself into the best possible position to use leverage to stretch a group of muscles. Many people sit on the ground with their legs spread wide apart, hoping to lean forward and place their heads on the ground in an attempt to stretch the back of their legs. But most are not successful, because sitting on the floor in this way causes their bodies to fall backward, and thus they are working against gravity. All they need to do to get great leverage in this movement is to assume the same position standing up. Standing with their legs spread wide apart and leaning forward, they can use the weight of their body to lean over and have great leverage to stretch the back of their legs, for gravity is now on their side instead of them fighting gravity. It's a humbling lesson about what is more powerful—gravity or us. The answer is obvious!

Remember that the best stretching occurs when you resist while moving through the greatest possible range of motion, starting from the muscle being as short as possible and moving to where the muscle is as long as possible. Remember, you can keep elongating the muscles you are stretching only if you can still resist the elongation. If you move into ranges of motion where the muscles cannot resist, you are not stretching—you are overstretching.

Insurance Against Pain

Again, the most surprising thing about using resistance is that it takes the pain out of stretching. If you do not resist, you will lose control and most likely injure yourself. In a sense, resistance protects the muscle from overextension. Unnecessary pain occurs when the range of motion exceeds the correct amount of resistance. Simply put, too great a range of motion with too little resistance equals pain. The most surprising thing about using resistance is that it takes the pain out of traditional stretching. A muscle that is being stretched must be able to contract maximally throughout that muscle's entire stretch length in order to become truly flexible. Taking your body into optimal ranges of motion without simultaneously and maximally resisting results in overstretching and sometimes injury.

Key Questions When Using Resistance to Stretch

Do I need to warm up?

Yes. You can warm up by stringing together all sixteen different types of stretches into a nonstop aerobic flow. Many people feel that the best time to stretch is after they've finished an aerobic activity like swimming or biking, when they are heated deeply to their core. You definitely need to be very warmed up before you start stretching when using maximum resistance.

When do I start to resist and when do I stop?

You start to resist when you have gotten yourself in a position where the muscles you are about to stretch are as short as possible. You then resist and begin to elongate the muscles while continuing to resist. You stop when the muscles you are stretching can no longer resist.

What direction do I move into while resisting?

The general direction or path to move in is described for each stretch in the following stretching routine chapters. But you will find that you get the best stretch when you carefully feel the path that has the greatest resistance. Moving along this path of greatest resistance targets the tightest parts of the muscles. Not finding this path misses the best stretch.

At what speed do I move while stretching?

You need to move at all different speeds when you stretch, because that's how your muscles will be used. So sometimes you will move slowly, sometimes quite fast, and of course sometimes you will repose.

What range do I stretch into?

You can continue to lengthen muscles when you stretch only as long as they can resist the elongation. After a while you become pretty good at feeling the muscles that you are stretching contract, so you know if these muscles are continuing to contract.

How many repetitions should I do?

Consecutive reps of the same stretch are absolutely necessary to become flexible. Six to ten is usually a good number to do on each side per set. You need to do at least three sets to complete your stretch workout. But you should determine how many reps to perform by gauging your fatigue level. Repeating cycles of tension using resistance cause continual reflex releases in a muscle's length. Because you are contracting muscles, sooner or later they will tire. Stop before you get too fatigued. If you become too

fatigued, it takes the muscle twice as long to recover. So don't let yourself go too far, too fast.

How long should I resist?

When I stretch, it usually takes 15–60 seconds to do 6–10 reps of a stretch. But if you are isometrically resisting to get a stretch, then for some muscles, for some people, on some days, 8–15 seconds is a perfect amount of time to stay in a stretch. At other times, minutes of resistance are necessary to remove tenseness. Resist only as long as it feels good.

How hard should I resist?

Begin by resisting in a way that feels good and then gradually increase the resistance. The more intensely you resist, the shorter the period of time you'll be able to stay in the stretch. If you resist too hard, you will be unable to breathe naturally. Learn to use the right amount of resistance so that you do not impede your ability to breathe. Remember: When you stretch a muscle using resistance, the tension level is twice that of weight training.

When can I use maximum resistance?

To increase your flexibility, you must maximally resist. Of course, you should always begin stretching using submaximal resistance, but once you've warmed up, you must do 6–10 reps of all stretches using maximal resistance to remove chronic past damage and tension in your body, and to facilitate continuous increases in your flexibility. Using maximum resistance takes time and practice to learn, but the results speak for themselves. After you've exercised and your body is warmed up is a great time to use maximum resistance.

How do previously injured muscles need to be stretched?

Previously injured muscles have scar tissue and additional layers of tough connective tissue around the injured area. These areas require special attention to correct. Injured areas require more reps, more sets, and more resistance to "clear" them and bring them into greater levels of performance than they had before they were injured. See Chapter 15.

Is too much resistance counterproductive?

As your stretching improves, you will discover that the better you are at using maximal resistance—whether moving or holding a stretch—the greater your gains. However, a note of caution is necessary here. As an eager beginner, you might make the mistake of equating pain with progress. Resisting

too long, too hard, or too often is counterproductive. Learn to listen to your body. It will tell you when you are pushing (or resisting) too much. If you can't breathe when resisting, then you are resisting too hard.

Being Creative—Dismantling in Order to Rebuild

Stretching makes you aware of areas of tension in your body. At the same time, it places you in a position to have the best leverage to create and use resistance to remove that tenseness. Difficult versions of the same type of stretches expose you to deeper and deeper levels of stiffness and inflexibility, until the most advanced stretches bring you into positions that allow you to totally remove a chronic type of tenseness.

It might seem like a contradiction to use resistance to remove resistance. One way to better understand this is to look at its parallel in homeopathic medicine, called the Law of Similars. This principle states that substances that cause healthy people to get specific symptoms can cure diseases that have these same specific symptoms. In other words, "Like cures like." Recognized by physicians and philosophers since ancient times, this idea became the basis of homeopathy's founder Samuel Hahnemann's formulation of the homeopathic doctrine. Although it contradicted medical thinking at the time, which typically prescribed medicines that counteracted and suppressed the symptoms of an illness, Hahnemann used substances that were intended to mobilize the body's own self-healing powers to resist the illness.

Now that you know about the different ways to resist while stretching, let's try the stretches. They are organized in beginner, intermediate, assisted, and advanced series. There are sixteen in each series.

The Sixteen Stretches

Part Three

Chapter 9

Sixteen Essential Stretches and the Stretching (and Strengthening) Routines

When the whole body hums

SOMETIMES YOU JUST HAVE TO TAKE one big free fall into the pool, submerging yourself from head to toe, to get the full effect of an experience. This chapter gives you a full-body plunge into the waters of resistance stretching. You will discover the power of all sixteen different stretches. I call these the "magic sixteen."

Many years have passed since I first discovered the power of resistance stretching and developed the sixteen types of stretches for the whole body. You can stretch all eight meridian-muscle groups in your lower body and eight meridian-muscle groups in your upper body, one after the other, and literally feel your body start to hum.

After you have learned each of the individual stretches, I teach you how to combine the sixteen stretches in one session. The order of the stretches is similar to the order of the energy flow in TCM.

Your Body and the Sixteen Essential Stretches

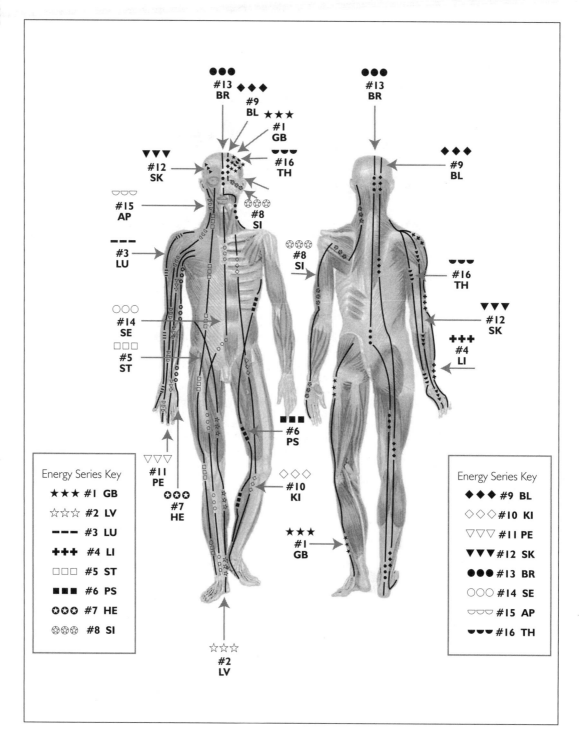

Energy Series Key

★★★ #1 GB
☆☆☆ #2 LV
–––– #3 LU
+++ #4 LI
□□□ #5 ST
■■■ #6 PS
✪✪✪ #7 HE
✿✿✿ #8 SI

Energy Series Key

◆◆◆ #9 BL
◇◇◇ #10 KI
▽▽▽ #11 PE
▼▼▼ #12 SK
●●● #13 BR
○○○ #14 SE
◡◡◡ #15 AP
▬▬▬ #16 TH

Don't leave out any of the stretches. You need to feel the satisfaction of having every muscle in your body stretched at one time. Have fun!

You will find that certain stretches from each routine are easier for you to do than others. I have designed resistance stretching so that once you become familiar with the individual stretches, you can select stretches that challenge you the way you want. You can move from beginner to advanced with the routines that I have created, or incorporate stretches from each of the routines into a personalized flow series that is beneficial for your whole body.

- **Energy series 1: Beginner stretches** Stretches that anyone can do, especially people who are just learning to stretch or are new at resistance stretching.
- **Energy series 2: Intermediate stretches** These stretches are for you to try only after you've learned and can easily perform the beginner resistance stretches.
- **Energy series 3: Assisted stretches** Assisted stretches require skilled stretchers who understand the limits and considerations that are necessary to ensure your safe development.
- **Energy series 4: Advanced stretches** Stretches for people who can comfortably do the intermediate stretches and have learned to resist maximally when stretching.

Once you've practiced the energy series for a while, it's time to begin tailoring your stretching routines to your own specifications. The next section offers four flex tests that will help you to design your own personal stretch routines based on your physical, spiritual, emotional, and psychological needs.

Chapter 10

Energy Series 1

Beginner stretch (and strength) series

1. Knee to Forehead (GB)

Start Stretch Here—Position 1.

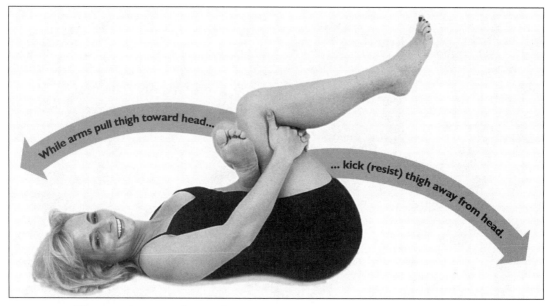

While arms pull thigh toward head...

... kick (resist) thigh away from head.

REMEMBER: The stretch occurs during the movement, not simply at the finishing position. So start resisting in position 1 and continuously resist while moving into position 2.

Getting Into This Stretch

Lie on your back. Pull your right knee halfway to your chest and place your left ankle over your right knee. Place both hands on the back of your right thigh.

Adding Resistance While Stretching

Stretch the muscles on the side of your left hip and leg by continuously resisting your left leg and ankle against your right thigh, as you pull your right knee toward your chest and forehead with your arms. Strengthen these same muscles by using your left leg and ankle to push your right thigh away from you, as your arms resist. Repeat both the stretching and strengthening movements 6–10 times, then change sides.

Finish Stretch Here—Position 2.

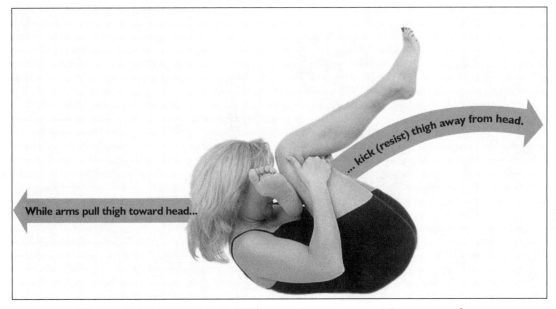

REMEMBER: Keep resisting in position 2. Without resistance, you won't get a stretch.

Breathing

Inhale as you get into the starting position. Exhale as you move through the stretch.

Benefits

This stretch can help to increase the flexibility and strength of your lateral leg, torso, neck, and head muscles, improve the health of your gallbladder and tendons, improve your fat metabolism, and improve your ability to turn from side to side. Psychologically, this stretch can help to increase your devotion to others, help you to be more decisive, help you to step up to the plate when the going gets tough, and can help to dismantle dependency problems.

2. Lateral Bend (LV)

Start Stretch Here—Position 1.

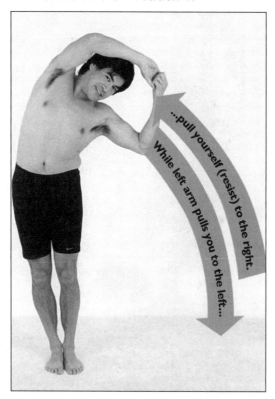

...pull yourself (resist) to the right.

While left arm pulls you to the left...

REMEMBER: The stretch occurs during the movement, not simply at the finishing position. So start resisting in position 1 and continuously resist while moving into position 2.

Getting Into This Stretch

Stand with your feet together and grasp your hands together above your head.

Adding Resistance While Stretching

Continuously contract the muscles on the left side of your torso that you are about to stretch by pulling your left arm downward and using your right arm to lean over to the left; turn your torso and head up toward the ceiling. Return to the starting position. Repeat 6–10 times, then change sides.

Finish Stretch Here—Position 2.

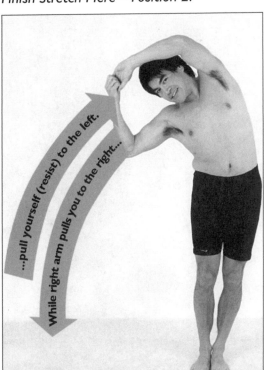

...pull yourself (resist) to the left.

While right arm pulls you to the right...

REMEMBER: Keep resisting in position 2. Without resistance, you won't get a stretch.

Breathing

Inhale as you get into the starting position. Exhale as you move through the stretch.

Benefits

This stretch can improve the health of your liver and tendons, help to detoxify your body, and improve your overall appearance.

Psychologically, this stretch increases your awareness of what you truly desire, helps you to become more helpful and less repressed, helps you to develop deeper independence, and can help to dismantle codependence.

3. Dip (LU)

Start Stretch Here—Position 1.

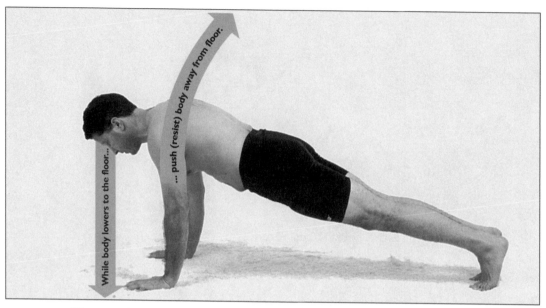

While body lowers to the floor...

... push (resist) body away from floor.

REMEMBER: The stretch occurs during the movement, not simply at the finishing position. So start resisting in position 1 and continuously resist while moving into position 2.

Getting Into This Stretch

Kneel on all fours, hips aligned over your knees and hands and wrists under and in alignment with your shoulders (this is the traditional push-up position). With your knees either on the ground or off, dip down, bringing your chest to the ground.

Adding Resistance While Stretching

Continuously contract the muscles you about to stretch on the front of your chest and the inside of your arms by resisting as you lower yourself into the push-up position. Return to starting position. Repeat 6–10 times.

Finish Stretch Here—Position 2.

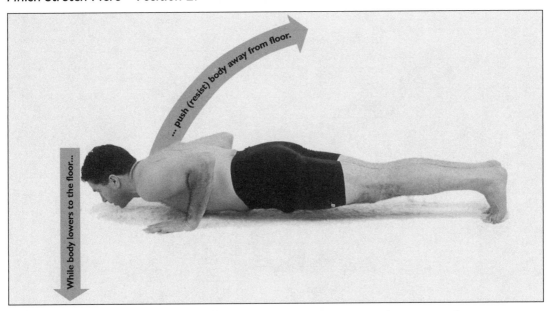

push (resist) body away from floor.

While body lowers to the floor...

REMEMBER: Keep resisting in position 2. Without resistance, you won't get a stretch.

Breathing

Inhale as you get into the stretch. Exhale as you move through the stretch.

Benefits

This stretch can improve the health of your lungs, increase the oxygen levels in your blood, improve your endurance, and increase your strength. Psychologically, this stretch can help to increase your personal power, help you develop better boundaries, and assist you in dismantling passive-aggressive behaviors.

4. Grapevine Arms (LI)

Start Stretch Here—Position 1.

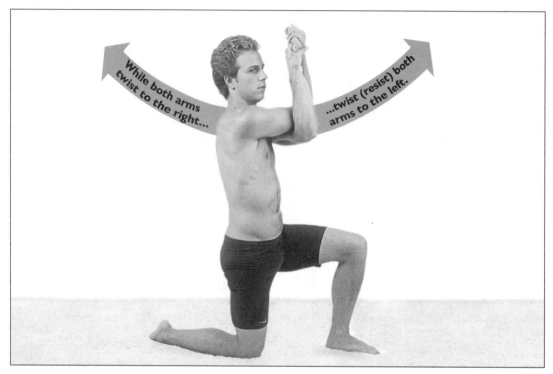

While both arms twist to the right...

...twist (resist) both arms to the left.

REMEMBER: The stretch occurs during the movement, not simply at the finishing position. So start resisting in position 1 and continuously resist while moving into position 2.

Getting Into This Stretch

Kneel on the floor. Lift your left arm up to the height of your shoulder. Cross your right arm over your left arm at the elbow, wrapping your right arm around your left. Interlock your forearms and hands.

Adding Resistance While Stretching

Continuously contract the muscles on the back of your left shoulder that you are about to stretch by pressing your left elbow sideways while your right hand pulls your left elbow across your chest. Push your elbows against each other and press your hands together. Return to starting. Repeat 6–10 times.

Finish Stretch Here—Position 2.

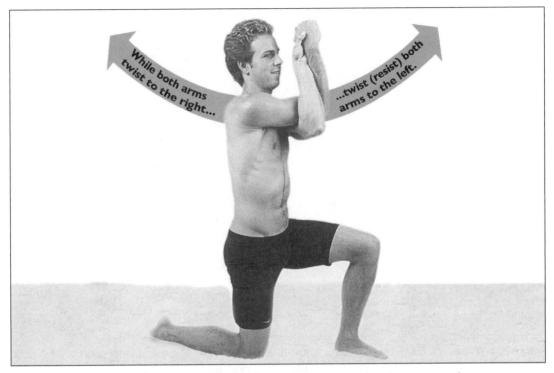

REMEMBER: Keep resisting in position 2. Without resistance, you won't get a stretch.

Breathing

Inhale as you get into the starting position. Exhale as you move through the stretch.

Benefits

This stretch can help to improve the health of your large intestine, venous blood flow, and bowel movements. Psychologically, this stretch increases your ambition, self-control, feelings of serenity, and fairness, and helps you dismantle obsessive-compulsive behaviors.

5. Thigh Stretch at Wall (ST)

Start Stretch Here—Position 1.

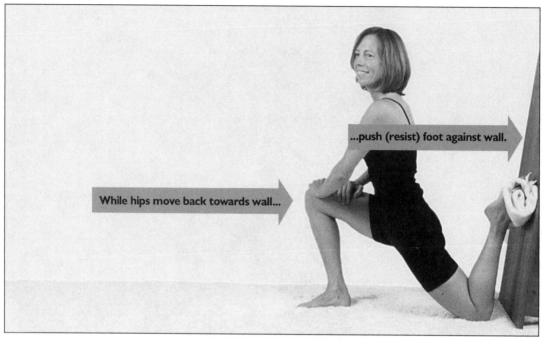

While hips move back towards wall...

...push (resist) foot against wall.

REMEMBER: The stretch occurs during the movement, not simply at the finishing position. So start resisting in position 1 and continuously resist while moving into position 2.

Getting Into This Stretch

Kneel on all fours with your hips aligned over your knees, and your hands and wrists under and in alignment with your shoulders. Bring your left lower leg and foot up against the wall (you can use a towel or small pillow to cushion your foot). Step up onto your right foot in front of you and lunge deeply forward, slanting your torso slightly forward.

Adding Resistance While Stretching

Continuously contract the muscles on the front of your left thigh that you are about to stretch by pushing against the wall with your left foot while you bring your hips back next to your left foot. Return to starting position. Repeat 6–10 times, then change sides.

Finish Stretch Here—Position 2.

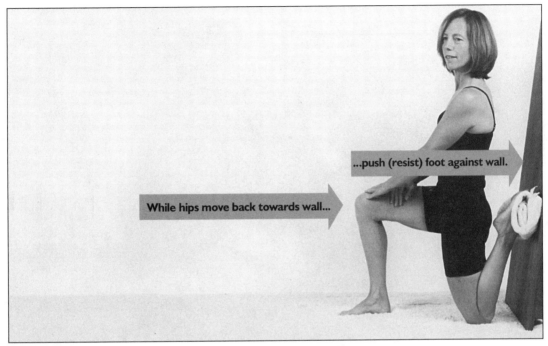

While hips move back towards wall...

...push (resist) foot against wall.

REMEMBER: Keep resisting in position 2. Without resistance, you won't get a stretch.

Breathing

Inhale as you get into the starting position. Exhale as you move through the stretch.

Benefits

This stretch can improve the health of your stomach and decrease or eliminate muscular pain. Psychologically, this stretch can help to increase your sobriety, self-expression, and self-realization; makes you more youthful, more entrepreneurial, more sympathetic; and helps you develop an exceptional taste for quality and a love for work and movement. This stretch can help you to dismantle addictions and eccentric behaviors.

6. Wide Leg Forward Bend (Standing or Seated) (PS)

Start Stretch Here—Position 1.

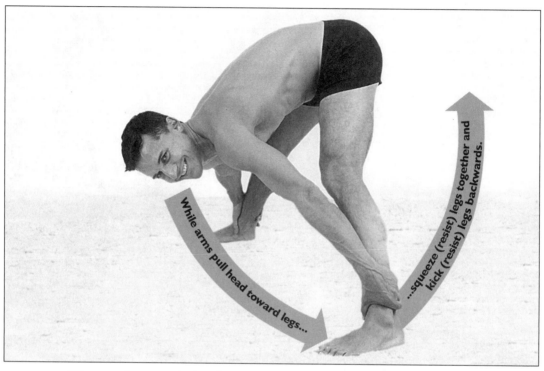

While arms pull head toward legs...

...squeeze (resist) legs together and kick (resist) legs backwards.

REMEMBER: The stretch occurs during the movement, not simply at the finishing position. So start resisting in position 1 and continuously resist while moving into position 2.

Getting Into This Stretch

Standing, spread your legs shoulder width apart or wider, and bend forward. Grasp your ankles with both hands.

Adding Resistance While Stretching

Continuously contract the muscles on the inside back of your thighs as you bend forward, straighten your legs, and pull your head between your legs with your arms. Repeat 6–10 times.

Finish Stretch Here—Position 2.

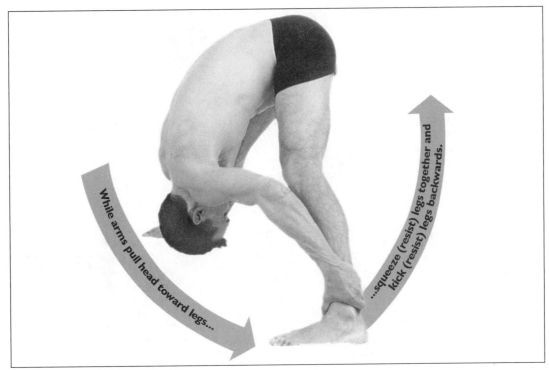

While arms pull head toward legs...

...squeeze (resist) legs together and kick (resist) legs backwards.

REMEMBER: Keep resisting in position 2. Without resistance, you won't get a stretch.

Breathing

Inhale as you get into the starting position. Exhale as you move through the stretch.

Benefits

This stretch can improve the health of your pancreas, thus improving your digestion, increase your energy, and decrease or eliminate fascia or scar tissue damage. Psychologically, this stretch can help to increase your temperance, empathy, and communication skills, and can help you become more playful. This stretch can assist you in dismantling indifference and move you away from a feeling of martyrdom.

7. Chair Pull-Down (HE)

Start Stretch Here—Position 1.

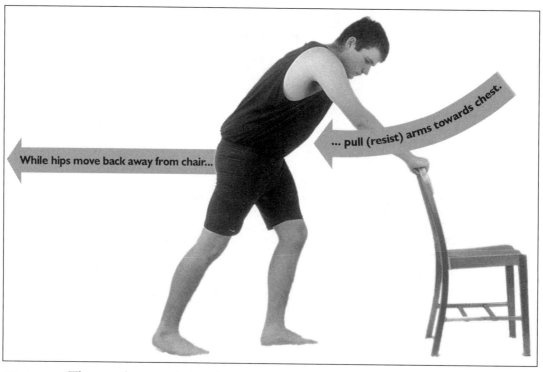

While hips move back away from chair...

... pull (resist) arms towards chest.

REMEMBER: The stretch occurs during the movement, not simply at the finishing position. So start resisting in position 1 and continuously resist while moving into position 2.

Getting Into This Stretch

Standing, face the back of a chair. Place both hands on the top of the chair next to each other. Stand in a lunge position with your left foot forward.

Adding Resistance While Stretching

Continuously contract your chest muscles and the muscles on the inside of your arms through your thumb as you begin to stretch by pulling downward with your arms as your head moves down between your arms. Return to the starting position and repeat 6–10 times.

Finish Stretch Here—Position 2.

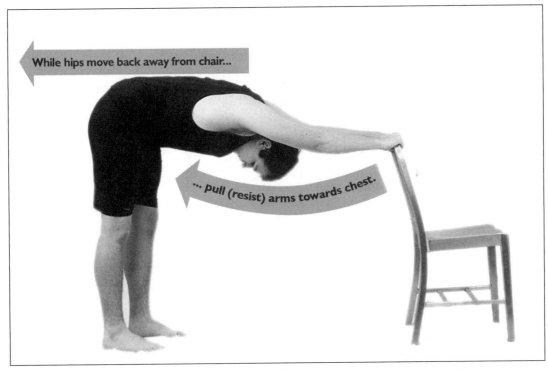

REMEMBER: Keep resisting in position 2. Without resistance, you won't get a stretch.

Breathing

Inhale as you get into the starting position. Exhale as you move through the stretch.

Benefits

This stretch can help to improve the health of your heart and blood flow. Psychologically, this stretch can increase your wakefulness and your ability to be unconditionally loving and joyful, improve your mediation skills, help you know when to take action, and help you keep momentum on projects. This stretch can also help to dismantle your sloth and avoidance.

8. Infinity (SI)

Start Stretch Here—Position 1.

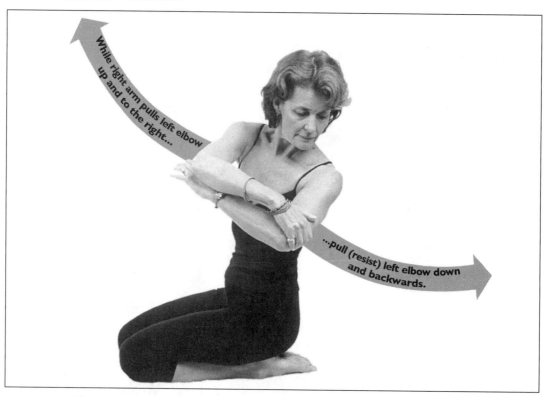

While right arm pulls left elbow up and to the right...

...pull (resist) left elbow down and backwards.

REMEMBER: The stretch occurs during the movement, not simply at the finishing position. So start resisting in position 1 and continuously resist while moving into position 2.

Getting Into This Stretch

Sit on the floor, lift your arms to chest level. Place the palm of your right hand at the bend of the opposite elbow and rest your right elbow on the top of your left hand.

Adding Resistance While Stretching

Continuously contract the muscles on the back of your shoulder and arm that you are about to stretch as you pull your right elbow forward and circle your arms through a figure eight or an infinity pattern. Each hand should push against each elbow. Repeat 6–10 times, then switch sides.

Finish Stretch Here—Position 2.

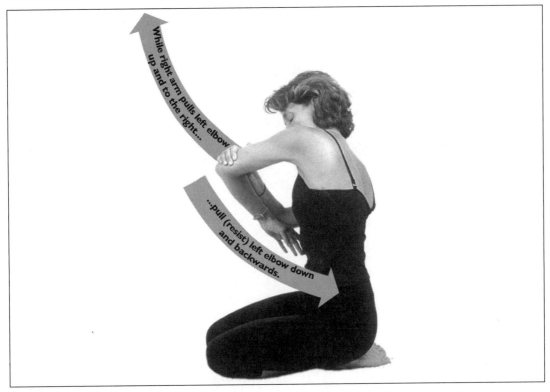

REMEMBER: Keep resisting in position 2. Without resistance, you won't get a stretch.

Breathing

Inhale as you get into the starting position. Exhale as you move through the stretch.

Benefits

This stretch can improve the health of your small intestine and increase cerebrospinal fluid movement up your spine. Psychologically, this stretch can make you more creative, passionate, and romantic, and can help you to dismantle depression.

9. Central Leg Extension (BR)

Start Stretch Here—Position 1.

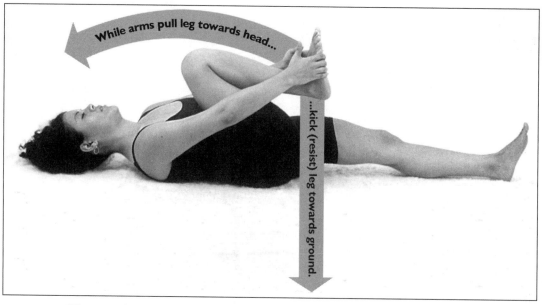

While arms pull leg towards head...

...kick (resist) leg towards ground.

REMEMBER: The stretch occurs during the movement, not simply at the finishing position. So start resisting in position 1 and continuously resist while moving into position 2.

Getting Into This Stretch

Lie on the floor on your back. Bring your right knee up to your chest and bend your lower leg. Grasp hold of your right ankle and foot with both hands.

Adding Resistance While Stretching

Contract the muscles you are about to stretch on the back of your legs and up your spine by kicking your heel toward your butt while you bring your heel up toward your head with your hands. Repeat 6–10 times. Switch sides.

Finish Stretch Here—Position 2.

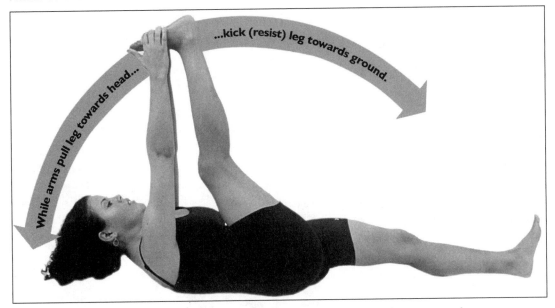

While arms pull leg towards head...

...kick (resist) leg towards ground.

REMEMBER: Keep resisting in position 2. Without resistance, you won't get a stretch.

Breathing

Inhale as you get into the starting position. Exhale as you move through the stretch.

Benefits

This stretch can help to improve the health of your brain and central nervous system. Psychologically, this stretch can help to increase your ability to master whatever you are doing, help you to be more trusting, and can help you to dismantle feelings of paranoia.

10. Hip Flexor Stretch (SE)

Start Stretch Here—Position 1.

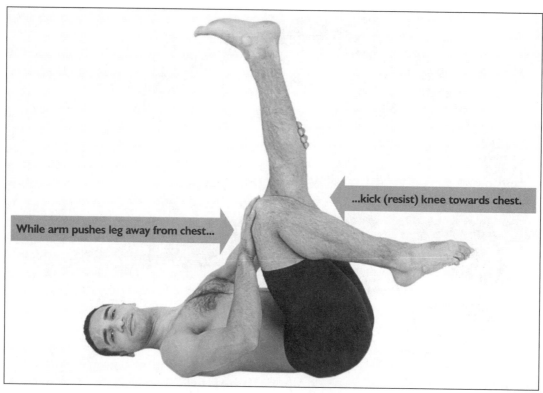

While arm pushes leg away from chest...

...kick (resist) knee towards chest.

REMEMBER: The stretch occurs during the movement, not simply at the finishing position. So start resisting in position 1 and continuously resist while moving into position 2.

Getting Into This Stretch

Lie on your back. Lift your left leg straight up and place it against the wall at a doorway (or hold the back of your left thigh with your left hand as vertically as possible but with your hips remaining on the ground). Bring your right knee up to your chest.

Adding Resistance While Stretching

Contract the muscles you are about to stretch on the front of your right hip as you push your left leg against the wall (or against your hand) while pushing your right knee away from you. Return to the starting position and repeat 6–10 times. Change sides.

Finish Stretch Here—Position 2.

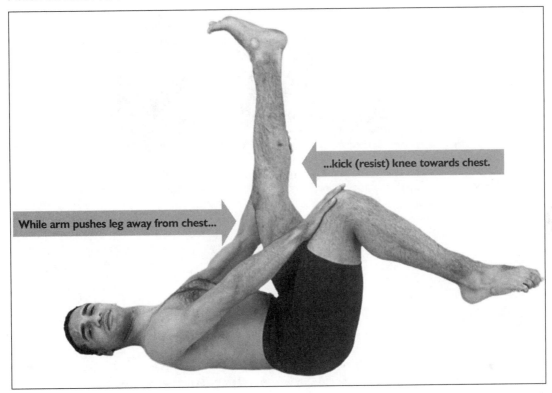

While arm pushes leg away from chest...

...kick (resist) knee towards chest.

REMEMBER: Keep resisting in position 2. Without resistance, you won't get a stretch.

Breathing

Inhale as you get into the starting position. Exhale as you move through the stretch.

Benefits

This stretch can help to improve the health of your sexual organs and endocrine functions, increase your gracefulness, and improve your looks. Psychologically, this stretch teaches you to be more caring and more accepting of yourself and can help to dismantle your bad moods.

11. Lightning on the Floor (PE)

Start Stretch Here—Position 1.

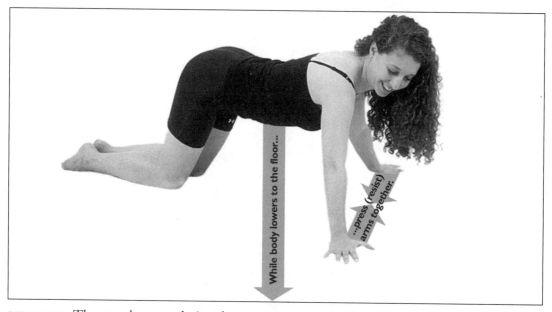

While body lowers to the floor...

...press (resist) arms together.

REMEMBER: The stretch occurs during the movement, not simply at the finishing position. So start resisting in position 1 and continuously resist while moving into position 2.

Getting Into This Stretch

Go onto all fours. Place your arms close to one another with your palms against the floor.

Adding Resistance While Stretching

Contract the muscles you are about to stretch on the center front of your chest, arms, and palms as you press your arms together and slide your arms sideways until your chest is on the floor. Return to the starting position and repeat 6–10 times.

Finish Stretch Here—Position 2.

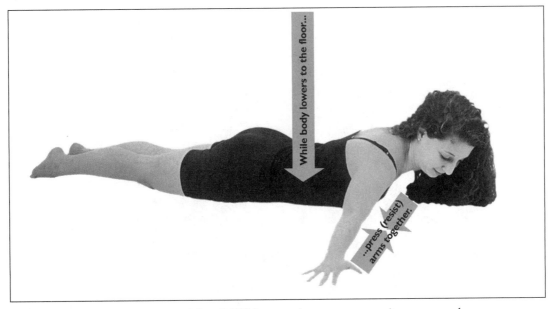

While body lowers to the floor...

...press (resist) arms together.

REMEMBER: Keep resisting in position 2. Without resistance, you won't get a stretch.

Breathing

Inhale as you get into the starting position. Exhale as you move through the stretch.

Benefits

This stretch can help to improve the health of your pericardium and circulation to your hands, feet, and genitals. Psychologically, this stretch can help you to be open-minded, ethical, judicious, philanthropic, and benevolent; it can help to improve your sexual imagination, and it can help to dismantle self-defeating, self-sabotaging behaviors.

12. Child Pose (SK)

Start Stretch Here—Position 1.

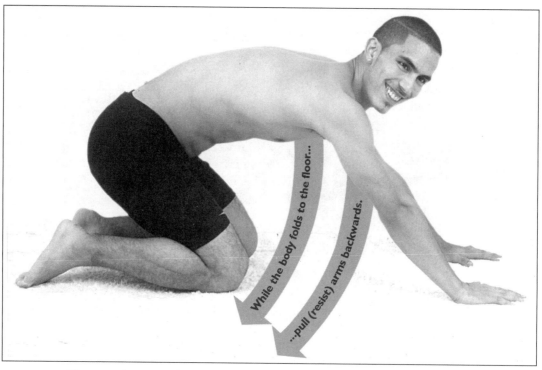

While the body folds to the floor...

...pull (resist) arms backwards.

REMEMBER: The stretch occurs during the movement, not simply at the finishing position. So start resisting in position 1 and continuously resist while moving into position 2.

Getting Into This Stretch

Kneel on the floor. Curl your torso and head toward your knees and place your elbows and hands parallel on the floor in front of you (the traditional sphinx position).

Adding Resistance While Stretching

Contract the muscles you are about to stretch on the back side of shoulders and arms as you pull backward and push downward against the floor. Press your lower legs against the floor as you arch like a snake. Repeat the resistance 6–10 times.

Finish Stretch Here—Position 2.

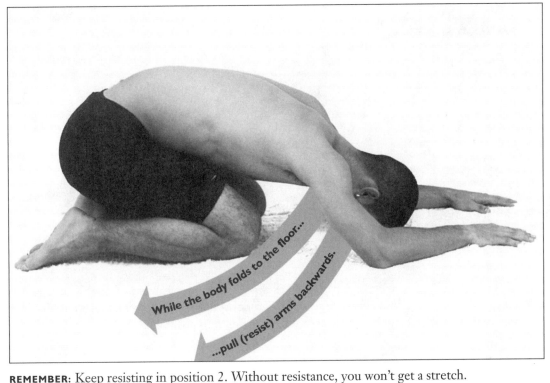

While the body folds to the floor...

...pull (resist) arms backwards.

REMEMBER: Keep resisting in position 2. Without resistance, you won't get a stretch.

Breathing

Inhale as you get into the starting position. Exhale as you move through the stretch.

Benefits

This stretch can help to improve the health of your skin and external immune system. Psychologically, this stretch can teach you to better handle stress, increase your cooperativeness, and help you rest. This stretch can help to dismantle antisocial behavior.

13. Crossover Leg Extension (BL)

Start Stretch Here—Position 1.

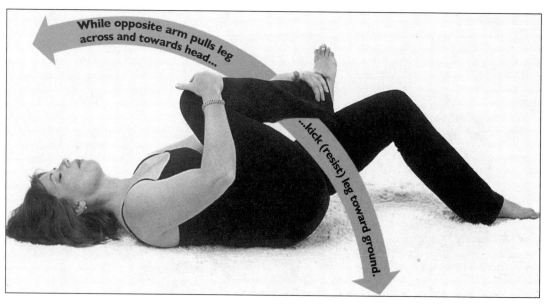

While opposite arm pulls leg across and towards head...

...kick (resist) leg toward ground.

REMEMBER: The stretch occurs during the movement, not simply at the finishing position. So start resisting in position 1 and continuously resist while moving into position 2.

Getting Into This Stretch

Lie on your back. Bring one knee toward your chest and grasp the outside of the foot with your opposite hand. (This stretch can be done lying on your back, seated, or standing.)

Adding Resistance While Stretching

Continuously contract the muscles along the back outside of your thigh that you are about to stretch by pulling your heel toward you as you lift your foot across you until your knee is as straight as possible. Repeat 6–10 times, then change sides.

Finish Stretch Here—Position 2.

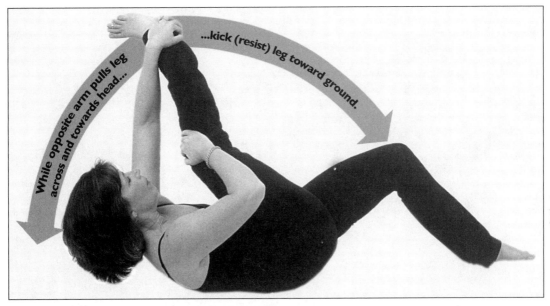

REMEMBER: Keep resisting in position 2. Without resistance, you won't get a stretch.

Breathing

Inhale as you get into the starting position. Exhale as you move through the stretch.

Benefits

This stretch can help to improve the health of your bladder and your bones, improve your balance, and eliminate many back pains. Psychologically, this stretch can help to make you more hopeful and results oriented, increases your self-esteem, and can help to dismantle narcissistic behaviors.

14. Lotus at Wall (KI)

Start Stretch Here—Position 1.

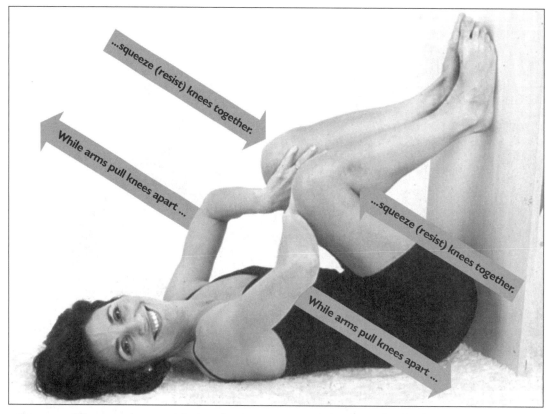

...squeeze (resist) knees together.

While arms pull knees apart ...

...squeeze (resist) knees together.

While arms pull knees apart ...

REMEMBER: The stretch occurs during the movement, not simply at the finishing position. So start resisting in position 1 and continuously resist while moving into position 2.

Getting Into This Stretch

Lie on your back with your hips close to the wall. Bend both knees and place the soles of your feet together on the wall.

Adding Resistance While Stretching

Continuously contract the muscles on the inside of your thighs that you are about to stretch by squeezing your thighs together while your hands open your knees sideways. Repeat 6–10 times.

Finish Stretch Here—Position 2.

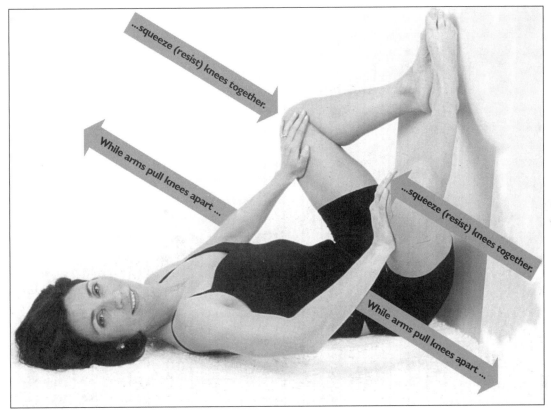

REMEMBER: Keep resisting in position 2. Without resistance, you won't get a stretch.

Breathing

Inhale as you get into the starting position. Exhale as you move through the stretch.

Benefits

This stretch can help to improve the health of your kidneys and joints. Psychologically, this stretch can give you greater understanding and confidence, and a better sense of humor. This stretch can also help you to become a better confidant and can help to dismantle "split" behaviors.

15. Locust at the Wall (AP)

Start Stretch Here—Position 1.

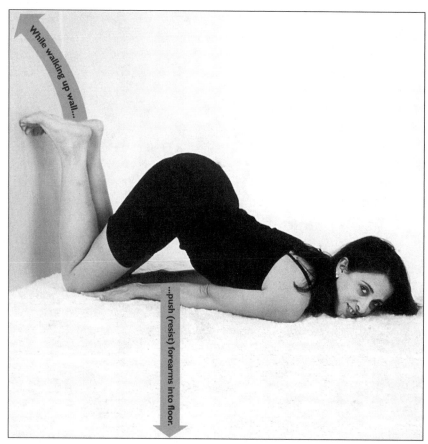

While walking up wall...

...push (resist) forearms into floor.

REMEMBER: The stretch occurs during the movement, not simply at the finishing position. So start resisting in position 1 and continuously resist while moving into position 2.

Getting Into This Stretch

Facing away from the wall, lie on your belly and place your hands under your hips with the palms down. You can use a strap to stabilize your hands.

Adding Resistance While Stretching

Contract the muscles you are about to stretch on the front of your arms by pressing your hands into the floor as you lean forward and balancing on the strap at your waist. Lift one leg at a time up onto the wall as high as you can. Stay balanced for several seconds. Return to the starting position and repeat 3 times.

Finish Stretch Here—Position 2.

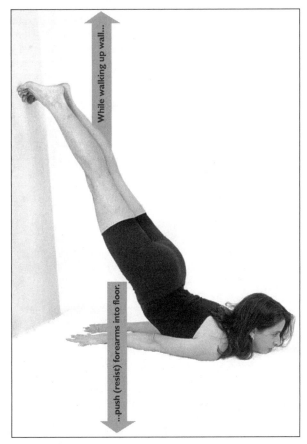

While walking up wall...

...push (resist) forearms into floor.

REMEMBER: Keep resisting in position 2. Without resistance, you won't get a stretch.

Breathing

Inhale as you get into the starting position. Exhale as you move through the stretch.

Benefits

This stretch can help to improve the health of your appendix and your cartilage, and help to detoxify your body. Psychologically, this stretch can help you to increase your ability to change and express gratitude, help to express your individuality, and can help to dismantle feelings of depersonalization.

16. Wall Roll-Down (TH)

Start Stretch Here—Position 1.

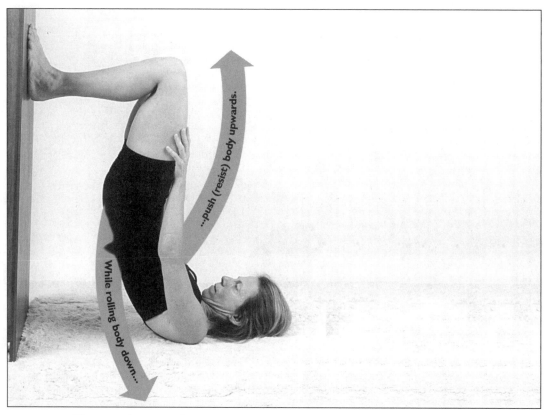

...push (resist) body upwards.

While rolling body down...

REMEMBER: The stretch occurs during the movement, not simply at the finishing position. So start resisting in position 1 and continuously resist while moving into position 2.

Getting Into This Stretch

Lie on your back with your hips close to the wall and both feet up on the wall, knees bent.

Adding Resistance While Stretching

Contract the muscles you are about to stretch on the back of your shoulders and back by pushing into the wall with both feet and pushing both hands into your thighs as you roll down your spine toward the floor. Return to the starting position and repeat 6–10 times.

Finish Stretch Here—Position 2.

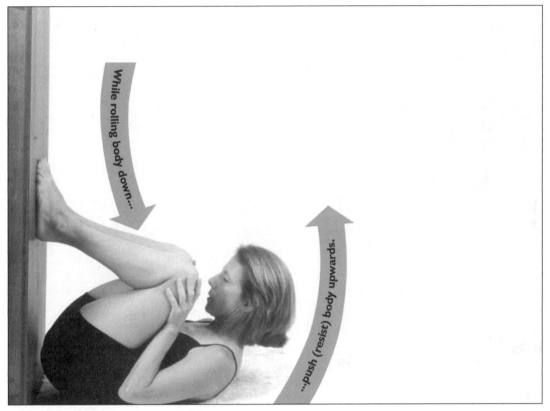

While rolling body down...

...push (resist) body upwards.

REMEMBER: Keep resisting in position 2. Without resistance, you won't get a stretch.

Breathing

Inhale as you get into the starting position. Exhale as you move through the stretch.

Benefits

This stretch can help to improve the health of your thymus, spleen, and internal immune system. Psychologically, this stretch can increase your ability to heal and forgive, increase your hospitality skills, and decrease feelings of distress, and can help to dismantle disease and brainwashing behaviors.

Chapter 11

Energy Series 2

Intermediate stretch (and strength) series

1. Rodeo (GB)

Start Stretch Here—Position 1.

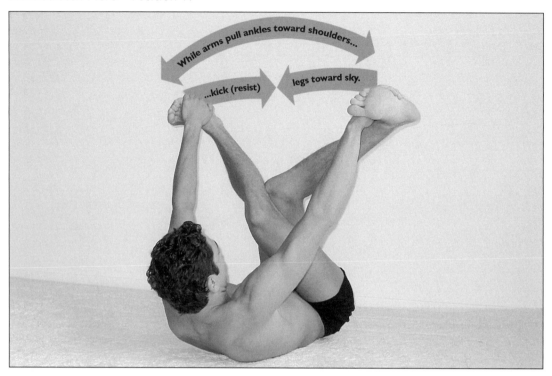

REMEMBER: The stretch occurs during the movement, not simply at the finishing position. So start resisting in position 1 and continuously resist while moving into position 2.

Getting Into This Stretch

Lie on your back. Bring your knees up to your chest, cross your legs at the knees, and grasp the outside of each ankle with each hand.

Adding Resistance While Stretching

Continuously contract the muscles on the sides of your left hip and leg by kicking your left lower leg up toward your hands. Then pull your ankles toward your shoulders. Return to the starting position. Repeat 6–10 times, then change sides.

Finish Stretch Here—Position 2.

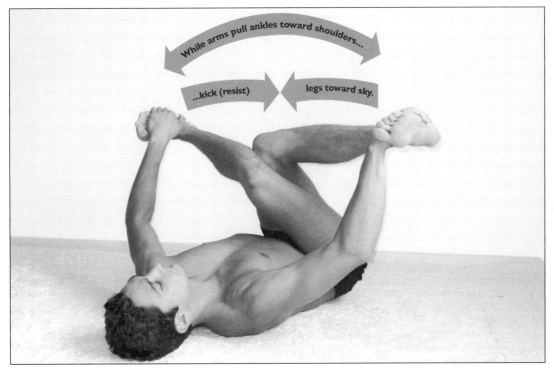

While arms pull ankles toward shoulders...

...kick (resist)

legs toward sky.

REMEMBER: Keep resisting in position 2. Without resistance, you won't get a stretch.

Breathing

Inhale as you get into position. Exhale as you move through the stretch.

Benefits

This stretch can help to improve the health of your gallbladder and tendons, your fat metabolism, and your ability to turn from side to side. Psychologically, this stretch can help to increase your devotion to others, help you to be more decisive, and help you to step up to the plate when the going gets tough. This stretch can help to dismantle dependency problems.

2. Sliding Side Split (LV)

Start Stretch Here—Position 1.

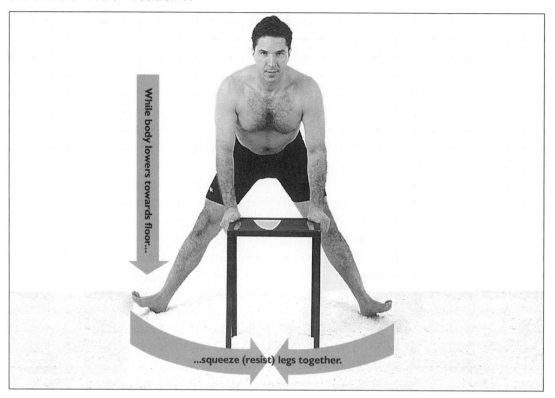

While body lowers towards floor...

...squeeze (resist) legs together.

REMEMBER: The stretch occurs during the movement, not simply at the finishing position. So start resisting in position 1 and continuously resist while moving into position 2.

Getting Into This Stretch

Stand with your legs spread. Place your hands on a chair in front of you.

Adding Resistance While Stretching

Continuously contract the muscles on the inside of both of your thighs that you are about to stretch by squeezing them toward each other as you slide your feet as wide apart as possible and flex your feet. Use your arms to help yourself raise out of the position. Return to the starting position. Repeat 6–10 times, then change sides.

Finish Stretch Here—Position 2.

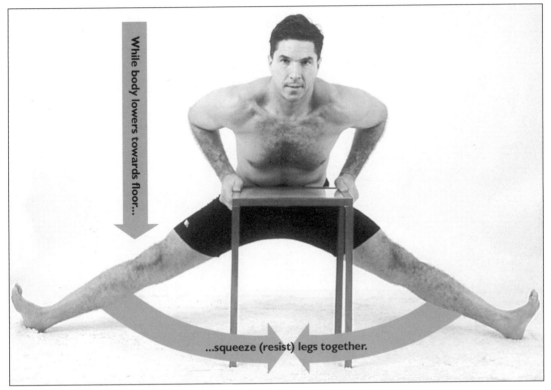

While body lowers towards floor...

...squeeze (resist) legs together.

REMEMBER: Keep resisting in position 2. Without resistance, you won't get a stretch.

Breathing

Inhale as you get into position. Exhale as you move through the stretch.

Benefits

This stretch can help to improve the health of your liver and tendons, detoxify your body, and improve your overall appearance. Psychologically, this stretch increases your awareness of what you truly desire, helps you to become more helpful and less repressed, helps you to develop deeper independence, and can help to dismantle codependency.

3. Handstand at the Wall (LU)

Start Stretch Here—Position 1.

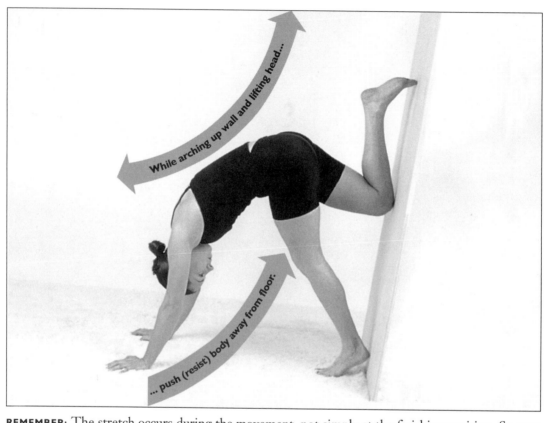

While arching up wall and lifting head...

... push (resist) body away from floor.

REMEMBER: The stretch occurs during the movement, not simply at the finishing position. So start resisting in position 1 and continuously resist while moving into position 2.

Getting Into This Stretch

Kneel on all fours with your backside facing the wall.

Adding Resistance While Stretching

Continuously contract the muscles you are about to stretch on the front of your chest and the inside of your arms by pressing your palms against the floor as you "walk" up the wall into a handstand. Lower one leg at a time. Return to starting position. Repeat 6–10 times.

Finish Stretch Here—Position 2.

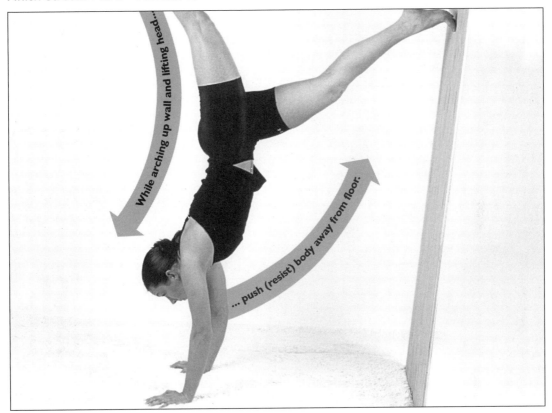

REMEMBER: Keep resisting in position 2. Without resistance, you won't get a stretch.

Breathing

Inhale as you get into position. Exhale as you move through the stretch.

Benefits

This stretch can help to improve the health of your lungs, increase the oxygen levels in your blood, improve your endurance, and increase your strength. Psychologically, this stretch can help to increase your personal power, help you to develop better boundaries, and assist you in dismantling passive-aggressive behaviors.

4. Kneeling Twist (LI)

Start Stretch Here—Position 1.

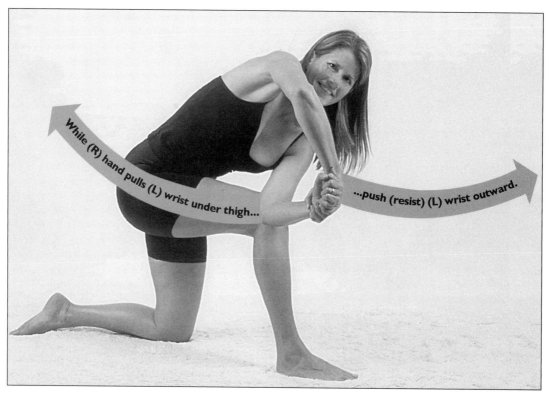

While (R) hand pulls (L) wrist under thigh...

...push (resist) (L) wrist outward.

REMEMBER: The stretch occurs during the movement, not simply at the finishing position. So start resisting in position 1 and continuously resist while moving into position 2.

Getting Into This Stretch

Kneel on the floor. Step out on your right foot with your right knee bent. Bend forward and place your left elbow on the outside of your right knee. Grasp your left wrist with your right hand.

Adding Resistance While Stretching

Continuously contract the muscles on the back of your left shoulder that you are about to stretch by pressing your left elbow against your right knee. Push your left arm outward while you pull it toward you with your right hand. Return to starting position. Repeat 6–10 times, then change sides.

Finish Stretch Here—Position 2.

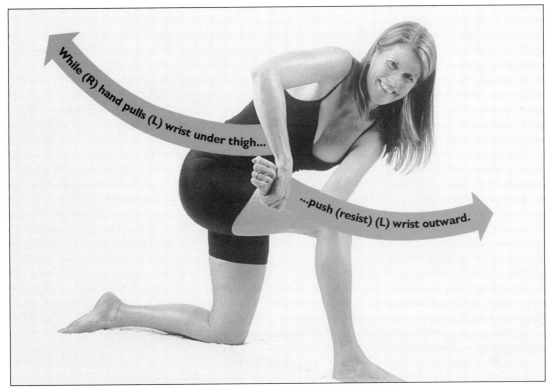

While (R) hand pulls (L) wrist under thigh...

...push (resist) (L) wrist outward.

REMEMBER: Keep resisting in position 2. Without resistance, you won't get a stretch.

Breathing

Inhale as you get into position. Exhale as you move through the stretch.

Benefits

This stretch can help to improve the health of your large intestine and venous blood flow and improve your bowel movements. Psychologically, this stretch increases your ambition, self-control, and feelings of serenity and fairness, and can help to dismantle obsessive-compulsive behaviors.

5. Kneeling Backbend (ST)

Start Stretch Here—Position 1.

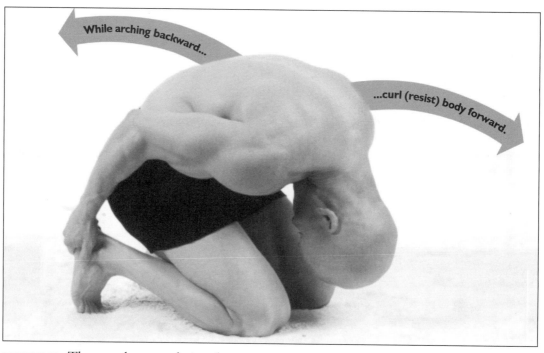

While arching backward...

...curl (resist) body forward.

REMEMBER: The stretch occurs during the movement, not simply at the finishing position. So start resisting in position 1 and continuously resist while moving into position 2.

Getting Into This Stretch

Kneel on the floor. Place both hands against the insides of your ankles; arch upward and backward.

Adding Resistance While Stretching

Continuously contract the muscles you are stretching on the front of your legs, torso, neck and head by (1) kicking your lower legs toward the floor, (2) pulling your knees up toward your chest, (3) curling your head, neck, and torso toward your waist; and (4) pressing your arms and hands outward against your ankles.

Finish Stretch Here—Position 2.

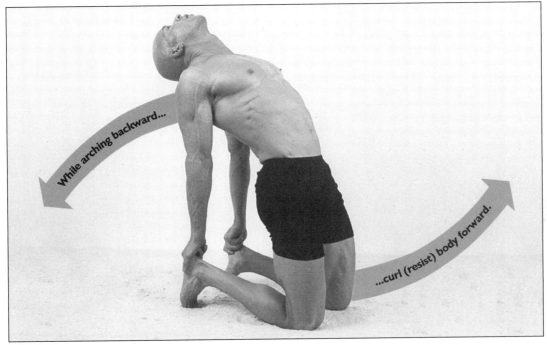

REMEMBER: Keep resisting in position 2. Without resistance, you won't get a stretch.

Breathing

Inhale as you get into position. Exhale as you move through the stretch.

Benefits

This stretch can help to improve the health of your stomach and muscles, and decrease or eliminate muscular pain. Psychologically, this stretch can help to increase your sobriety, self-expression, and self-realization; makes you more youthful, more entrepreneurial, and more sympathetic; and helps you develop exceptional taste for quality and a love for work and movement. This stretch can also help to dismantle addictions and eccentric behaviors.

6. Wide Leg Extension (PS)

Start Stretch Here—Position 1.

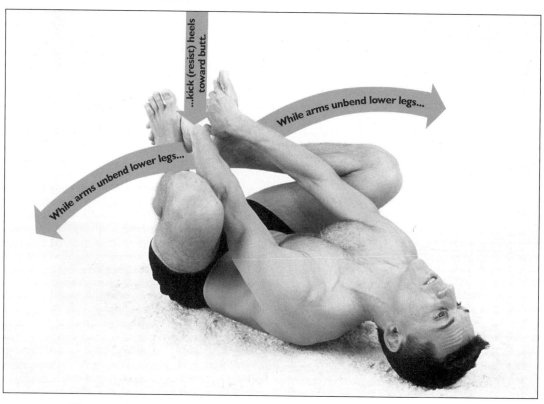

REMEMBER: The stretch occurs during the movement, not simply at the finishing position. So start resisting in position 1 and continuously resist while moving into position 2.

Getting Into This Stretch

Lie on your back with your legs wide open. Bend both knees and grasp the arch of each foot with each hand. (This stretch can be done while lying on your back or when seated.)

Adding Resistance While Stretching

Continuously contract the muscles on the inside back of your thighs that you are about to stretch by pulling your heels toward you as your hands straighten your legs upward and outward. Repeat 6–10 times.

Finish Stretch Here—Position 2.

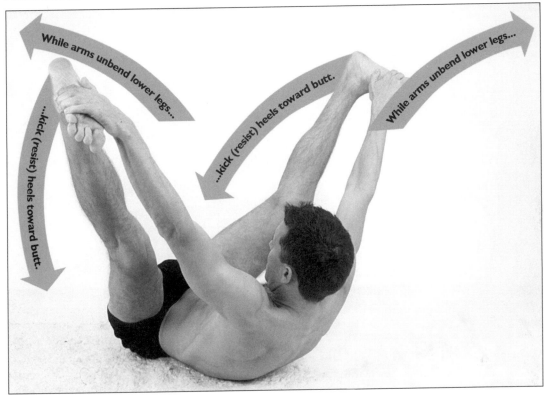

REMEMBER: Keep resisting in position 2. Without resistance, you won't get a stretch.

Breathing

Inhale as you get into position. Exhale as you move through the stretch.

Benefits

This stretch can help to improve the health of your pancreas, thus improving your digestion; increase your energy; decrease or eliminate fascia or scar tissue damage. Psychologically, this stretch can help to increase your temperance, empathy, and communication skills, and can help you become more playful. This stretch can assist you in dismantling indifference and move you away from feelings of martyrdom.

7. Forward Sliding (HE)

Start Stretch Here—Position I.

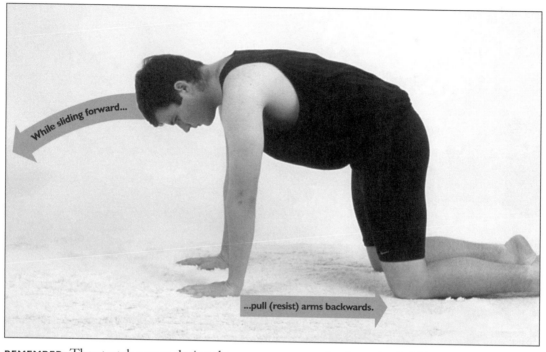

While sliding forward...

...pull (resist) arms backwards.

REMEMBER: The stretch occurs during the movement, not simply at the finishing position. So start resisting in position 1 and continuously resist while moving into position 2.

Getting Into This Stretch

Kneel on all fours.

Adding Resistance While Stretching

Continuously contract the muscles on the front of your chest and inside of your arms into your little fingers that you are about to stretch by pulling your arms down toward your waist but resisting by keeping them in place as you slide your body forward starting with the feet and extending the legs so that your hips are a few inches from the floor. Return to the starting position and repeat 6–10 times.

Finish Stretch Here—Position 2.

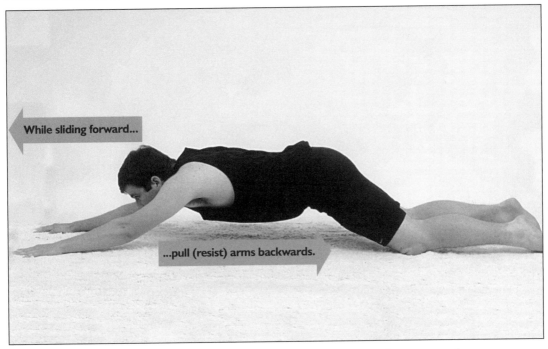

While sliding forward...

...pull (resist) arms backwards.

REMEMBER: Keep resisting in position 2. Without resistance, you won't get a stretch.

Breathing

Inhale as you get into position. Exhale as you move through the stretch.

Benefits

This stretch can help to improve the health of your heart and increase blood flow. Psychologically, this stretch can increase your wakefulness and your ability to be unconditionally loving and joyful, improve your mediation skills, help you know when to take action, and help you keep momentum on projects. This stretch can also help to dismantle your sloth and avoidance.

8. Gate Opener (SI)

Start Stretch Here—Position 1.

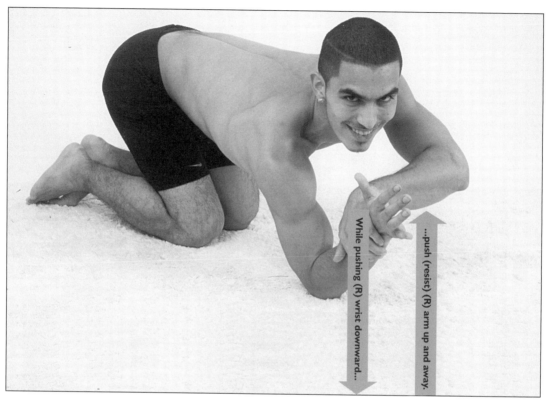

While pushing (R) wrist downward...

...push (resist) (R) arm up and away.

REMEMBER: The stretch occurs during the movement, not simply at the finishing position. So start resisting in position 1 and continuously resist while moving into position 2.

Getting Into This Stretch

Kneel on all fours. Place your right elbow on the floor in front of you and grasp the outside of your right wrist with your left hand.

Adding Resistance While Stretching

Continuously contract the muscles on the back of your shoulder and arm that you are about to stretch as you push your arm to the floor. Repeat this 6–10 times, then change sides.

Finish Stretch Here—Position 2.

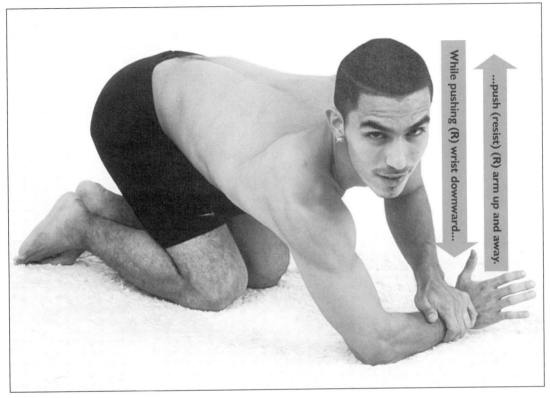

While pushing (R) wrist downward...

...push (resist) (R) arm up and away.

REMEMBER: Keep resisting in position 2. Without resistance, you won't get a stretch.

Breathing

Inhale as you get into position. Exhale as you move through the stretch.

Benefits

This stretch can help to improve the health of your small intestine and increase cerebrospinal fluid movement up your spine. Psychologically, this stretch can help to make you more creative, passionate, and romantic, and can help to dismantle depression.

9. Central Straight Leg Raise (With Strap) (BR)

Start Stretch Here—Position 1.

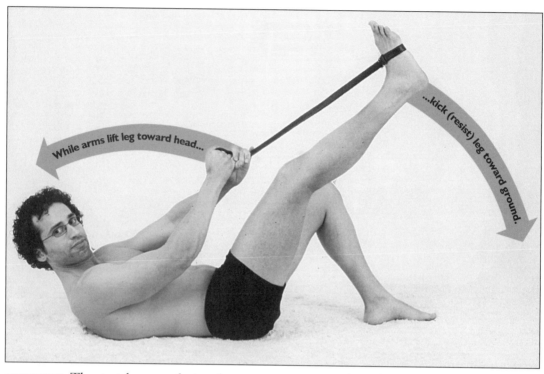

REMEMBER: The stretch occurs during the movement, not simply at the finishing position. So start resisting in position 1 and continuously resist while moving into position 2.

Getting Into This Stretch

Lie on your back and bend your knees. Attach a strap to your right foot, or grab your ankle or foot with both hands. (This stretch can be done lying on your back, seated, or standing.)

Adding Resistance While Stretching

Contract the muscles you are about to stretch on the back of your right leg by squeezing your thighs toward each other as you lift your right leg toward your head, pulling the leg up while your muscles push toward the ground. Return to the starting position and repeat 6–10 times. Change sides.

Finish Stretch Here—Position 2.

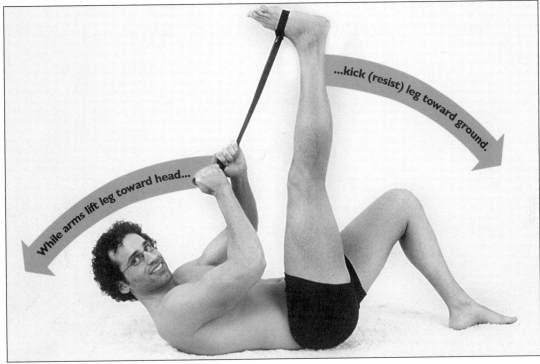

REMEMBER: Keep resisting in position 2. Without resistance, you won't get a stretch.

Breathing

Inhale as you get into position. Exhale as you move through the stretch.

Benefits

This stretch can help to improve the health of your brain and central nervous system. Psychologically, this stretch can help to increase your ability to master whatever you are doing, help you to be more trusting, and can help to dismantle feelings of paranoia.

10. Hip Flexor Lunge (SE)

Start Stretch Here—Position 1.

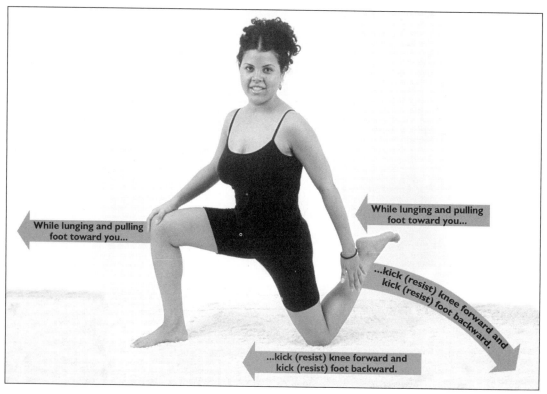

While lunging and pulling foot toward you...

While lunging and pulling foot toward you...

...kick (resist) knee forward and kick (resist) foot backward.

...kick (resist) knee forward and kick (resist) foot backward.

REMEMBER: The stretch occurs during the movement, not simply at the finishing position. So start resisting in position 1 and continuously resist while moving into position 2.

Getting Into This Stretch

Kneel on all fours; step out onto your right foot with your knee bent. Lift the lower part of the left leg and place your left hand on your left foot. Hold your left foot as you bring the foot to the back of your hip.

Adding Resistance While Stretching

Contract the muscles you are about to stretch on the front of your hip and thigh by lifting your lower left knee upward toward your shoulders, pushing your left foot against your left hand, as you lunge forward with your right knee. Return to the starting position. Repeat 6–10 times, then change sides.

Finish Stretch Here—Position 2.

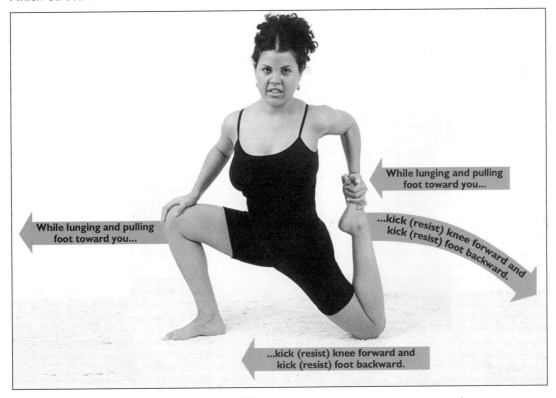

While lunging and pulling foot toward you...

While lunging and pulling foot toward you...

...kick (resist) knee forward and kick (resist) foot backward.

...kick (resist) knee forward and kick (resist) foot backward.

REMEMBER: Keep resisting in position 2. Without resistance, you won't get a stretch.

Breathing

Inhale as you get into position. Exhale as you move through the stretch.

Benefits

This stretch can help to improve the health of your sexual organs and endocrine functions, increase your gracefulness, and improve your looks. Psychologically, this stretch can help to teach you to be more caring and more accepting of yourself and can help to dismantle your bad moods.

11. Incline Plane Raise (PE)

Start Stretch Here—Position 1.

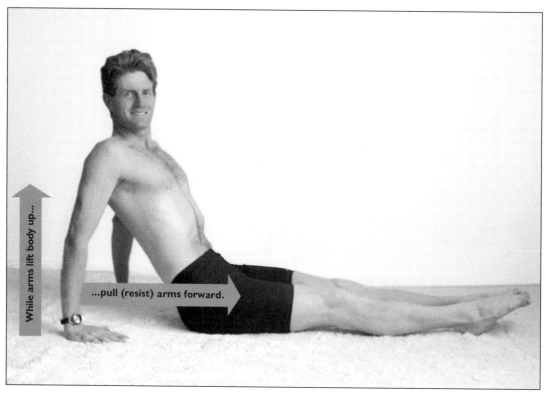

While arms lift body up...

...pull (resist) arms forward.

REMEMBER: The stretch occurs during the movement, not simply at the finishing position. So start resisting in position 1 and continuously resist while moving into position 2.

Getting Into This Stretch

Sit on the floor with your legs straight in front of you, toes pointed. Place your hands behind you, palms down, with your fingers pointing toward your body.

Adding Resistance While Stretching

Contract the muscles you are about to stretch on the center front of your chest, arms, and palms as you press yourself up into an inclined position. Lower your hips to the floor and return to the starting position. Repeat 6–10 times.

Finish Stretch Here—Position 2.

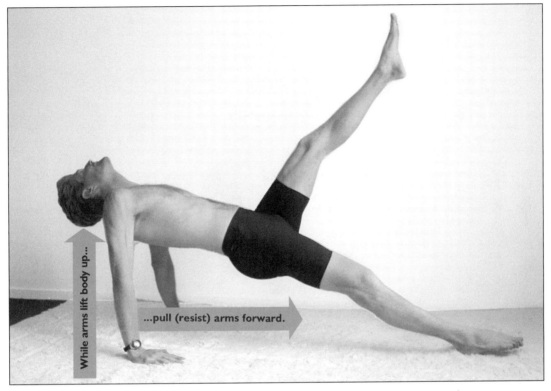

While arms lift body up...

...pull (resist) arms forward.

REMEMBER: Keep resisting in position 2. Without resistance, you won't get a stretch.

Breathing

Inhale as you get into position. Exhale as you move through the stretch.

Benefits

This stretch can help to improve the health of your pericardium, and increase circulation to your hands, feet, and genitals. Psychologically, this stretch can help you to be open-minded, ethical, judicious, philanthropic, and benevolent; improve your sexual imagination; and dismantle self-defeating, self-sabotaging behaviors.

12. Cobra Arch (SK)

Start Stretch Here—Position 1.

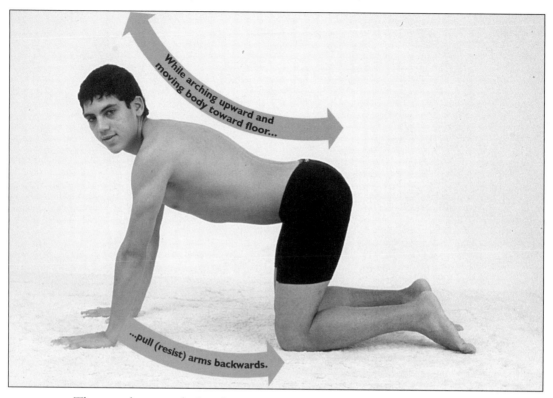

While arching upward and moving body toward floor...

...pull (resist) arms backwards.

REMEMBER: The stretch occurs during the movement, not simply at the finishing position. So start resisting in position 1 and continuously resist while moving into position 2.

Getting Into This Stretch

Lie prone: Place both hands parallel in front of you with your elbows bent and your forearms resting on the floor.

Adding Resistance While Stretching

Contract the muscles you are about to stretch on the back of your shoulders and arms, as you pull backward and push downward against the ground, raising into an arch. Press your lower legs against the ground. Repeat the resistance 6–10 times.

Finish Stretch Here—Position 2.

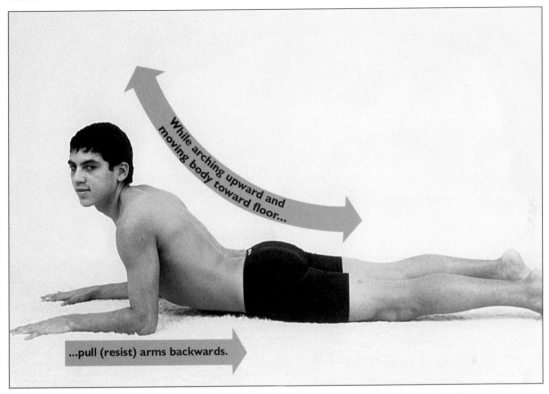

REMEMBER: Keep resisting in position 2. Without resistance, you won't get a stretch.

Breathing

Inhale as you get into position. Exhale as you move through the stretch.

Benefits

This stretch can help to improve the health of your skin and external immune system. Psychologically, this stretch can help you better handle stress, increase your cooperativeness, and help you rest. This stretch can help you to overcome antisocial behavior.

13. Crossover Straight Leg Stretch (With Strap) (BL)

Start Stretch Here—Position 1.

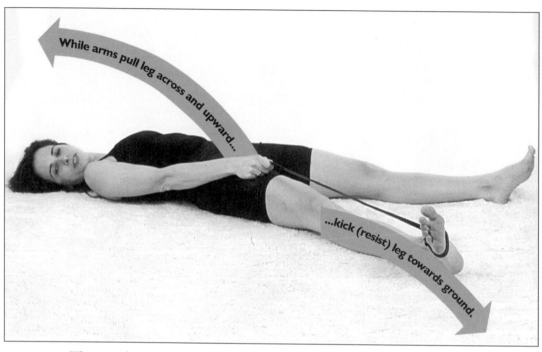

While arms pull leg across and upward...

...kick (resist) leg towards ground.

REMEMBER: The stretch occurs during the movement, not simply at the finishing position. So start resisting in position 1 and continuously resist while moving into position 2.

Getting Into This Stretch

Lie on your back and wrap a strap around the arch of your right foot. Open your right leg out to the side.

Adding Resistance While Stretching

Continuously contract the muscles along the back outside of your right thigh that you are about to stretch by pulling your right leg diagonally across your body up toward your left shoulder. Repeat 6–10 times, then change sides.

Finish Stretch Here—Position 2.

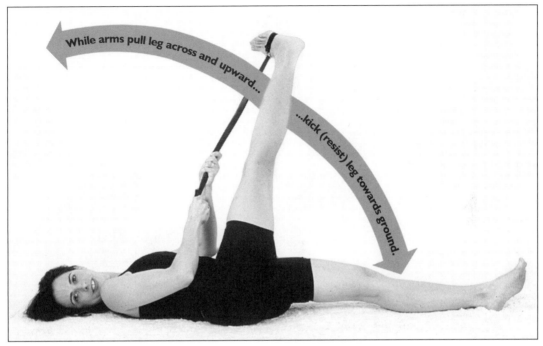

REMEMBER: Keep resisting in position 2. Without resistance, you won't get a stretch.

Breathing

Inhale as you get into position. Exhale as you move through the stretch.

Benefits

This stretch can help to improve the health of your bladder and bones, improve your balance, and eliminate many back pains. Psychologically, this stretch can help to make you more hopeful and results oriented, increase your self-esteem, and dismantle narcissistic behaviors.

14. Seated Lotus Opener (KI)

Start Stretch Here—Position 1.

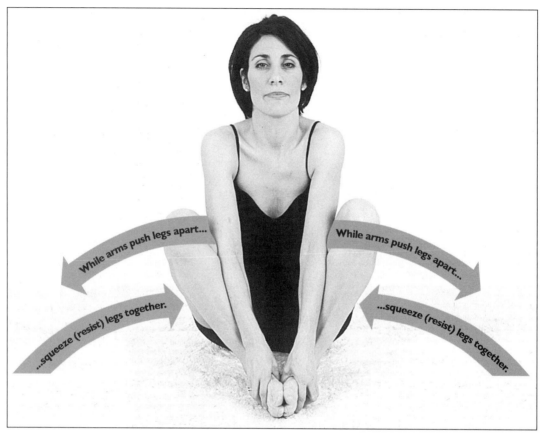

REMEMBER: The stretch occurs during the movement, not simply at the finishing position. So start resisting in position 1 and continuously resist while moving into position 2.

Getting Into This Stretch

Sit on the floor with your legs open, knees bent, and the soles of your feet together.

Adding Resistance While Stretching

Continuously contract the muscles on the inside of your thighs that you are about to stretch by squeezing your thighs together, while your hands or elbows press your knees toward the ground. Repeat 6–10 times.

Finish Stretch Here—Position 2.

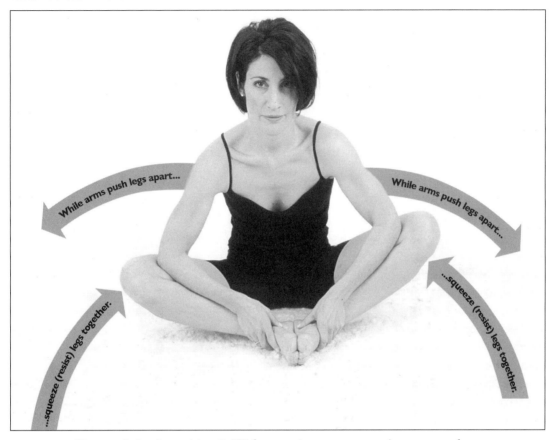

While arms push legs apart...

While arms push legs apart...

...squeeze (resist) legs together.

...squeeze (resist) legs together.

REMEMBER: Keep resisting in position 2. Without resistance, you won't get a stretch.

Breathing

Inhale as you get into position. Exhale as you move through the stretch.

Benefits

This stretch can help to improve the health of your kidneys and joints. Psychologically, this stretch can help to give you greater understanding and confidence, and a better sense of humor. This stretch can also help you to become a better confidant and can help to dismantle "split" behaviors.

149

15. Seesaw at Wall (AP)

Start Stretch Here—Position 1.

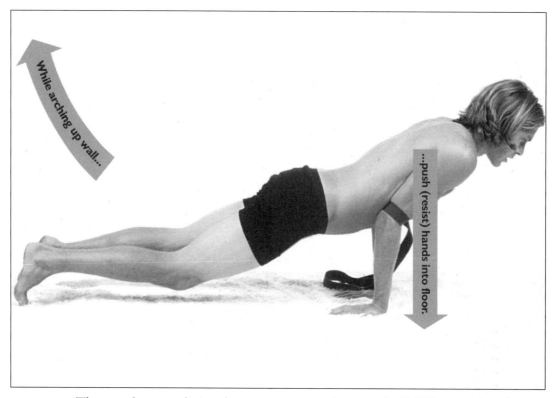

While arching up wall...

...push (resist) hands into floor.

REMEMBER: The stretch occurs during the movement, not simply at the finishing position. So start resisting in position 1 and continuously resist while moving into position 2.

Getting Into This Stretch

Kneel on the floor on all fours with your backside facing the wall and with your hands rotated with fingers pointing toward your body. Some people use a strap, as in the photo above, to encircle their arms to provide stability throughout this stretch.

Adding Resistance While Stretching

Contract the muscles you are about to stretch on the front of your arms by pressing your hands into the floor as you lean forward and balance on your elbows and as you "walk" up the wall as high as possible. Walk back down the wall. Return to the starting position and repeat 3 times.

Finish Stretch Here—Position 2.

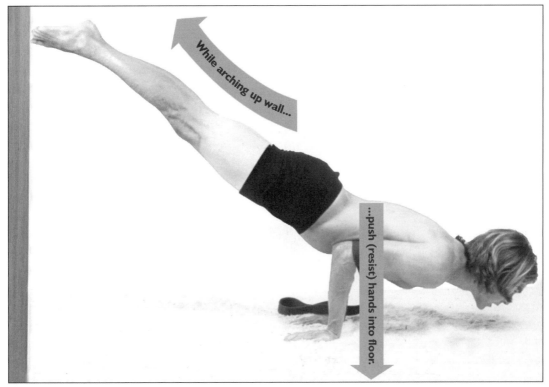

While arching up wall...

...push (resist) hands into floor.

REMEMBER: Keep resisting in position 2. Without resistance, you won't get a stretch.

Breathing

Inhale as you get into position. Exhale as you move through the stretch.

Benefits

This stretch can help to improve the health of your appendix and cartilage, and help to detoxify your body. Psychologically, this stretch can help you to increase your ability to change and express gratitude, help you to express your individuality, and can help to dismantle your feelings of depersonalization.

16. Backward Dip (TH)

Start Stretch Here—Position 1.

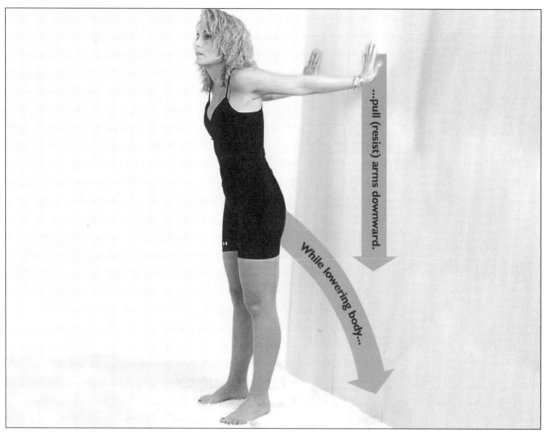

...pull (resist) arms downward.

While lowering body...

REMEMBER: The stretch occurs during the movement, not simply at the finishing position. So start resisting in position 1 and continuously resist while moving into position 2.

Getting Into This Stretch

Stand and face away from a wall. Place the palms of both hands against the wall as high as possible, with fingers pointing upward.

Adding Resistance While Stretching

Contract the muscles you are about to stretch on the back of your shoulders and back by pulling downward against the wall while keeping your hands in place, as you squat deeply. Return to the starting position and repeat 6–10 times.

Finish Stretch Here—Position 2.

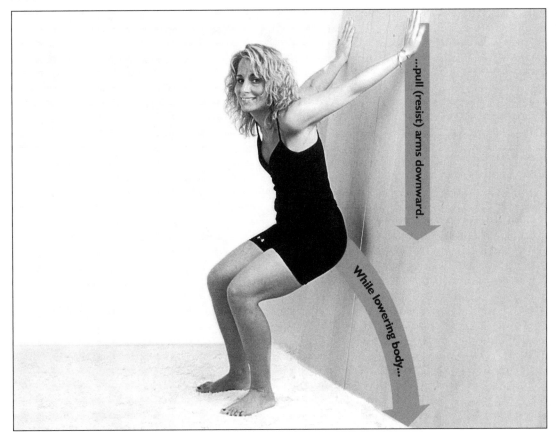

...pull (resist) arms downward.

While lowering body...

REMEMBER: Keep resisting in position 2. Without resistance, you won't get a stretch.

Breathing

Inhale as you get into position. Exhale as you move through the stretch.

Benefits

This stretch can help to improve the health of your thymus, spleen, and internal immune system. Psychologically, this stretch can help to increase your ability to heal and forgive, increase your hospitality skills, decrease feelings of distress, and can help to dismantle disease and brainwashing behaviors.

Chapter 12

Energy Series 3

Assisted stretch (and strength) series

HERE ARE SOME THINGS THAT ARE ESSENTIAL to know **when you are being assisted:**

- Besides stretching yourself, one or more other people can assist you. In many cases, being assisted increases your flexibility much faster than stretching by yourself. It is helpful to have someone else objectively analyze your stretch movements and where you are tight, which can be difficult for you to do on your own.

- Do not allow the person who is assisting you to take you farther than you want to go. Keep your own sense of authority about your body and always communicate with the person assisting you. Tell her when you want to start and stop and when the range, speed, force, and direction of the stretch feel right. She will have her own ideas, but it is important that you both come to the same conclusions about your stretch. Remember to show your appreciation and enjoy yourselves.

Here are some things that are essential to know **when you are assisting someone else:**

- You are moving the person through the stretch while he resists. It is very helpful if you give him feedback about what you discover while you assist him. For example, tell him where he is tight, how one side of his body compares to the other, or how his strength compares to his flexibility for each muscle group and movement. Don't underestimate how valuable your observations can be. You are outside, and he is inside! Being able to compare his feelings about himself and his stretches with what you tell him is priceless.
- Take the person into a range of motion where she can continue to resist maximally. Move at a speed that feels best to her and start and stop when she is ready. Decide how many reps and sets to do based on her

strength and fatigue. Avoid exhausting her. If you bring her to exhaustion, it takes the muscles three times as long to recover than if you stay within her limits.

- Guard against injury. The person being stretched can generate enormous amounts of force. His force may overcome your strength, in which case, you can possibly become injured. Sometimes it takes several people to assist someone; for example, when you stretch the hamstrings or other strong muscles. Make sure your leverage is optimal by carefully positioning yourself in a direct line with his movement and resistance. When you have good leverage, it should be relatively easy to overcome his resistance. If he is still overpowering you, either have him reduce his resistance or get more people to help.
- Because much more force is being used when you assist someone, I highly recommend that you "smash" those muscle groups you stretched so that you can help speed up the removal of the waste products produced from intense stretching. "Smashing" someone's hamstrings, gluteals, and calves can easily take a half hour or more. Keep "smashing" the muscles until they feel "peachy."
- As a rule of thumb, when you are stretching a particular group of muscles in someone else, the same group of muscles is being strengthened in you. If she can overpower you while you are stretching her, then those same muscles are being strained in you.

Err on the side of caution. You are at as big a risk of being injured as the person being stretched.

There is much more to know about assisting and being assisted than I've hinted at here. If you are going to be spending time regularly being assisted or assisting others, hire a certified meridian flexibility trainer, attend one of our workshops on learning how to assist, and buy *The Meridian Flexibility Teacher's Manual* through our Web site or at a workshop.

1. Assisted Thigh Crossover (GB)

Start Stretch Here—Position 1.

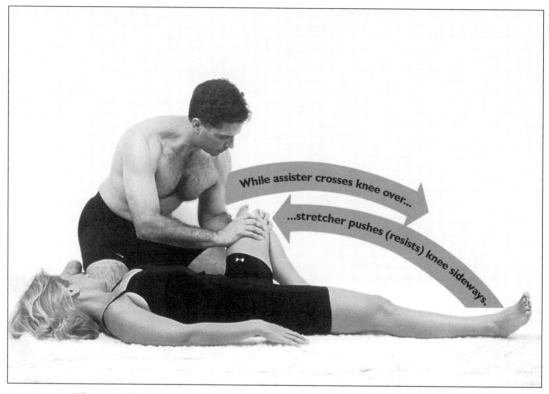

While assister crosses knee over...

...stretcher pushes (resists) knee sideways.

REMEMBER: The stretch occurs during the movement, not simply at the finishing position. So start resisting in position 1 and continuously resist while moving into position 2.

Getting Into This Stretch

Lie on your back on the floor. Bend your left knee, open your knee sideways, and place your left foot on the ground about 6 inches from your knee. The assister kneels next to you on your left side and places both hands on the outside of your knee.

Adding Resistance While Stretching

Contract the muscles you are about to stretch on the side of your hips and legs by pushing your knee sideways into the hands of the person assisting you. He will push your knee across your hips and torso as you resist. Return to the starting position. Repeat 6–10 times.

Finish Stretch Here—Position 2.

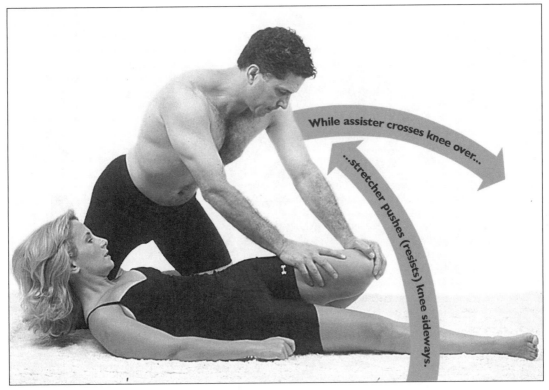

REMEMBER: Keep resisting in position 2. Without resistance, you won't get a stretch.

Breathing

Inhale as you get into the starting position. Exhale as you move through the stretch.

Benefits

This stretch can help to improve the health of your gallbladder and tendons, increase fat metabolism, and improve your ability to turn from side to side. This stretch can help to increase your devotion to others and help you to step up to the plate when the going gets tough, while helping to dismantle self-doubt and dependency problems.

2. Assisted Sideward Thigh Opener (LV)

Start Stretch Here—Position 1.

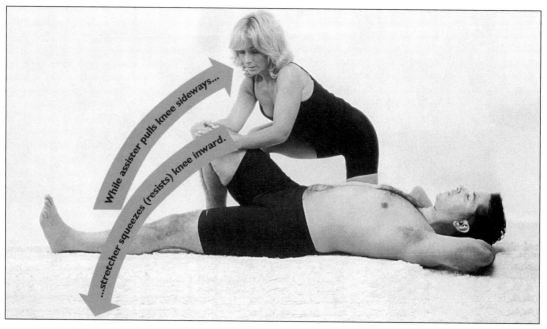

While assister pulls knee sideways...

...stretcher squeezes (resists) knee inward.

REMEMBER: The stretch occurs during the movement, not simply at the finishing position. So start resisting in position 1 and continuously resist while moving into position 2.

Getting Into This Stretch

Lie on your back on the floor with your legs extended. Bend your right knee. Keeping your knees together, place your right foot on the ground about 6 inches from your knee. The person assisting you kneels next to you on your right side and places both hands on the inside of your knee.

Adding Resistance While Stretching

Continuously contract the muscles on the inside of your right thigh that you are about to stretch by pushing your right thigh against the hands of the person assisting you, as she opens and pulls your right thigh sideways. Repeat 6–10 times. Return to the starting position and change sides.

Finish Stretch Here—Position 2.

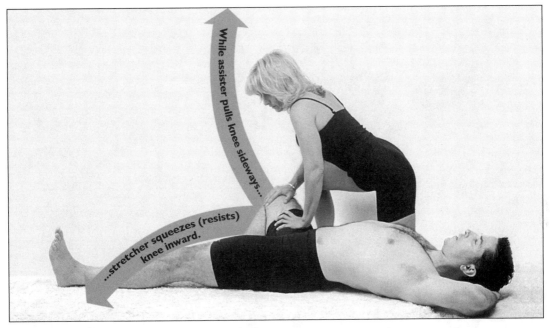

REMEMBER: Keep resisting in position 2. Without resistance, you won't get a stretch.

Breathing

Inhale as you get into the starting position. Exhale as you move through the stretch.

Benefits

This stretch can help to improve the health of your liver and tendons, detoxify you, and improve your overall appearance. Psychologically, this stretch increases your awareness of what you truly desire, helps you to become more helpful and less repressed, and helps you to develop deeper independence while dismantling codependency.

3. Assisted Reverse Throwing (LU)

Start Stretch Here—Position 1.

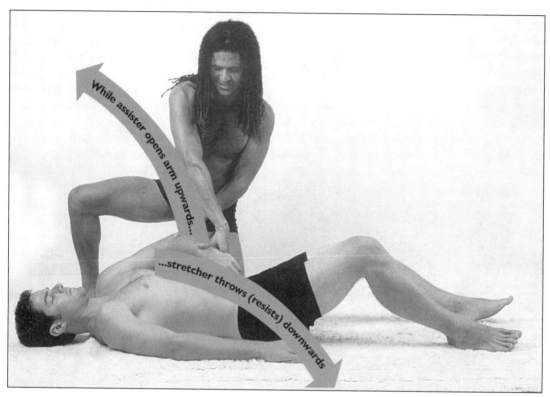

While assister opens arm upwards...

...stretcher throws (resists) downwards

REMEMBER: The stretch occurs during the movement, not simply at the finishing position. So start resisting in position 1 and continuously resist while moving into position 2.

Getting Into This Stretch

Lie on your back and slightly bend both knees while placing your feet on the floor. Lift your left arm across your body, bend your elbow, and allow the person assisting you to grasp your left wrist and elbow.

Adding Resistance While Stretching

Continuously contract the muscles you are about to stretch on the front of your chest and the inside of your arms by pressing against the hands of the person assisting you as she opens your arm upward and outward. Repeat 6–10 times. Return to the starting position and then switch sides.

Finish Stretch Here—Position 2.

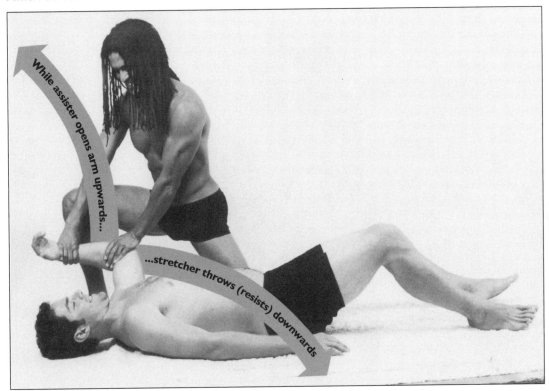

While assister opens arm upwards...

...stretcher throws (resists) downwards

REMEMBER: Keep resisting in position 2. Without resistance, you won't get a stretch.

Breathing

Inhale as you get into the starting position. Exhale as you move through the stretch.

Benefits

This stretch can help to improve the health of your lungs, increase oxygen levels in your blood, improve your endurance, and increase your strength. Psychologically, this stretch can help to increase your personal power, develop better boundaries, and dismantle passive-aggressive behaviors.

4. Assisted Grapevine Arms (LI)

Start Stretch Here—Position 1.

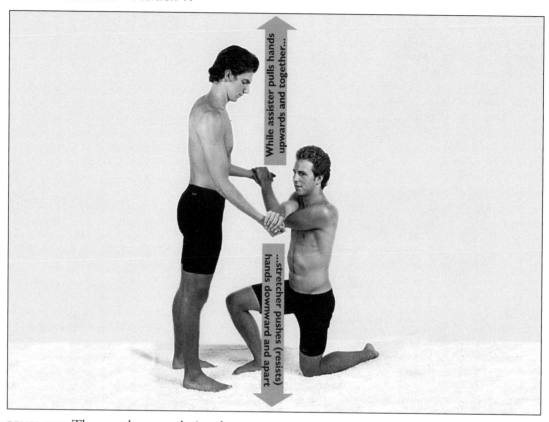

While assister pulls hands upwards and together...

...stretcher pushes (resists) hands downward and apart

REMEMBER: The stretch occurs during the movement, not simply at the finishing position. So start resisting in position 1 and continuously resist while moving into position 2.

Getting Into This Stretch

Kneel with both knees on the floor. Lift your right knee and place your foot on the floor about 6 inches in front of you. Lift your arms toward your head, cross your upper arms over one another, and clasp the hands of the person assisting you.

Adding Resistance While Stretching

Continuously contract the muscles on the back of your shoulders that you are about to stretch by pressing your hands downward and away from each other as the person assisting you lifts and twists your arms together.

Finish Stretch Here—Position 2.

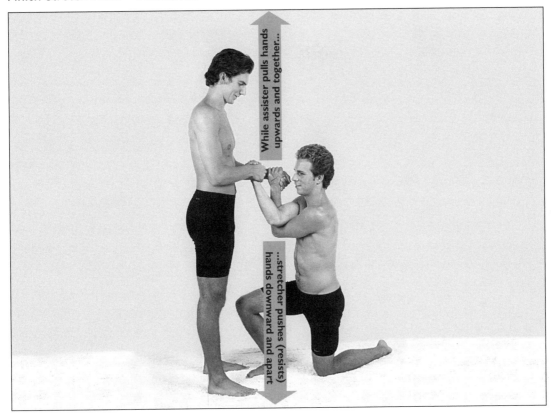

While assister pulls hands upwards and together...

...stretcher pushes (resists) hands downward and apart

REMEMBER: Keep resisting in position 2. Without resistance, you won't get a stretch.

Breathing

Inhale as you get into the starting position. Exhale as you move through the stretch.

Benefits

This stretch can help to improve the health of your large intestine, increase venous blood flow, and improve your bowel movements. Psychologically, this stretch can help to increase your ambition, self-control, feelings of serenity and fairness while helping to dismantle obsessive-compulsive behaviors.

5. Assisted Backbend With Bench (ST)

Start Stretch Here—Position 1.

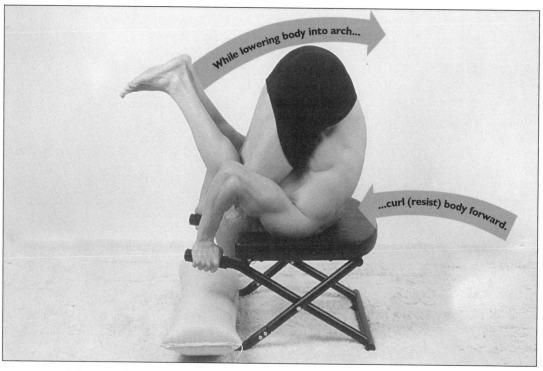

While lowering body into arch...

...curl (resist) body forward.

REMEMBER: The stretch occurs during the movement, not simply at the finishing position. So start resisting in position 1 and continuously resist while moving into position 2.

Getting Into This Stretch

Using a backbend bench, grab hold of the handles, place both knees on the bench, and curl up into a ball.

Adding Resistance While Stretching

Continuously contract the muscles you are stretching on the front of your legs, torso, neck and head by (1) pulling your lower legs toward your hips; (2) pulling your knees up toward your chest; (3) curling your head, neck, and torso toward your waist; and (4) pulling your arms and hands against the handles while you slowly uncurl and bring your feet to the floor.

Finish Stretch Here—Position 2.

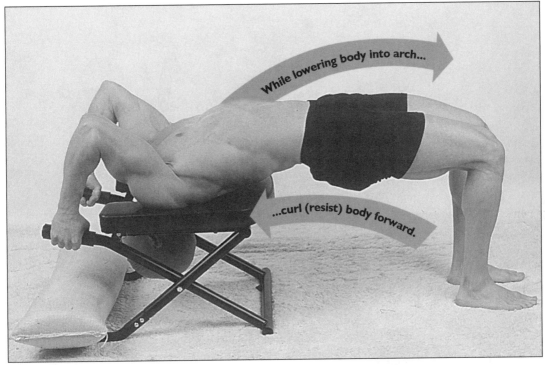

While lowering body into arch...

...curl (resist) body forward.

REMEMBER: Keep resisting in position 2. Without resistance, you won't get a stretch.

Breathing

Inhale as you get into the starting position. Exhale as you move through the stretch.

Benefits

This stretch can help to improve the health of your stomach and decrease or eliminate muscular pain. Psychologically, this stretch can help to increase your sobriety, self-expression, and self-realization; makes you more youthful, entrepreneurial, and sympathetic; helps you to develop exceptional taste for quality and a love for work and movement; and can help to dismantle addictions and eccentric behaviors.

6. Assisted Spleen Arms (PS)

Start Stretch Here—Position 1.

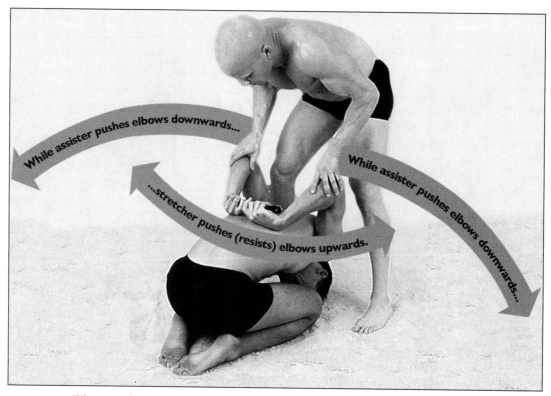

REMEMBER: The stretch occurs during the movement, not simply at the finishing position. So start resisting in position 1 and continuously resist while moving into position 2.

Getting Into This Stretch

Kneel in a child pose. Using a strap to connect your hands for stability, place your hands behind your mid- or upper back.

Adding Resistance While Stretching

Continuously contract the muscles on the inside back of your shoulders as you resist the movement of the person assisting you, who lowers and lifts your arms by holding them just below the elbow. Repeat 6–10 times.

Finish Stretch Here—Position 2.

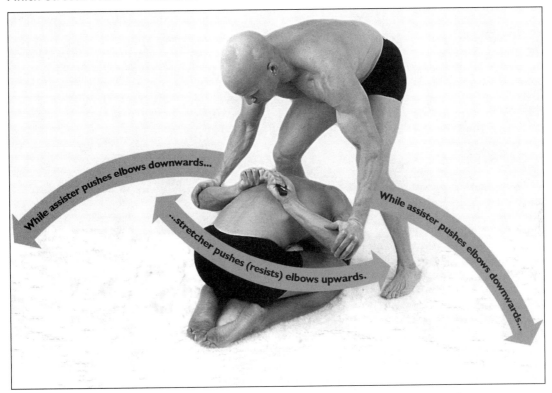

REMEMBER: Keep resisting in position 2. Without resistance, you won't get a stretch.

Breathing

Inhale as you get into the starting position. Exhale as you move through the stretch.

Benefits

This stretch can help to improve the health of your pancreas, thus improving your digestion; increase your energy; and decrease or eliminate fascia or scar tissue damage. Psychologically, this stretch can help to increase your temperance, empathy, and communication skills; helps you become more playful; and can help to dismantle indifference and martyrdom.

7. Assisted Back Lying Arm Pull-Downs (HE)

Start Stretch Here—Position 1.

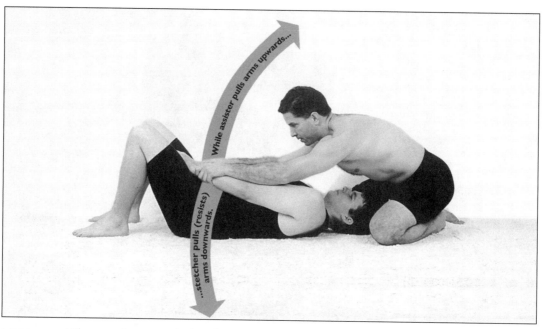

While assister pulls arms upwards...

...stetcher pulls (resists) arms downwards.

REMEMBER: The stretch occurs during the movement, not simply at the finishing position. So start resisting in position 1 and continuously resist while moving into position 2.

Getting Into This Stretch

Lie on your back and place your palms against your inner thighs. The person assisting you will kneel just above your head and grasp your wrists.

Adding Resistance While Stretching

Continuously contract the muscles on the front of your chest and the inside of your arms through to your little fingers that you are about to stretch by pushing your arms downward as the person assisting you lifts your arms above your head. Remain in the stretch for 1–2 minutes or longer while continuously resisting.

Finish Stretch Here—Position 2.

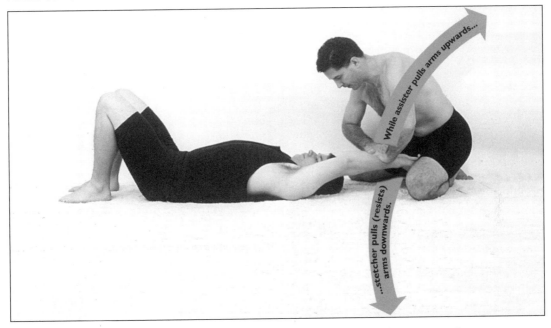

REMEMBER: Keep resisting in position 2. Without resistance, you won't get a stretch.

Breathing

Inhale as you get into the starting position. Exhale as you move through the stretch.

Benefits

This stretch can help to improve the health of your heart and blood flow. Psychologically, this stretch helps to increase your wakefulness, improve your ability to be unconditionally loving and joyful and to take the right action at the right time. It also helps you to keep the momentum going on projects, improves your mediation skills, and helps to dismantle your sloth and avoidance.

8. Assisted Arm Crossover (SI)

Start Stretch Here—Position 1.

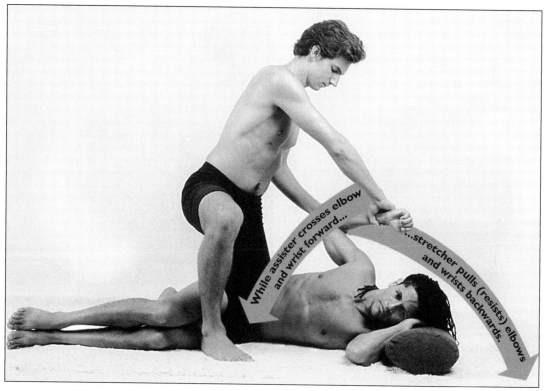

While assister crosses elbow and wrist forward...

...stretcher pulls (resists) elbows and wrists backwards

REMEMBER: The stretch occurs during the movement, not simply at the finishing position. So start resisting in position 1 and continuously resist while moving into position 2.

Getting Into This Stretch

Lie on the floor on your left side with both knees slightly bent. The person assisting you kneels behind your hip and crosses you by placing his right foot on the floor in front of you. Your assister holds your right wrist with his right hand and holds your elbow with his left hand.

Adding Resistance While Stretching

Continuously contract the muscles on the back of your right shoulder and arm as you pull your right elbow backward as the person assisting you crosses and pushes your right arm in front of your chest and down to the floor. Repeat 6–10 times. Return to the starting position and change sides.

Finish Stretch Here—Position 2.

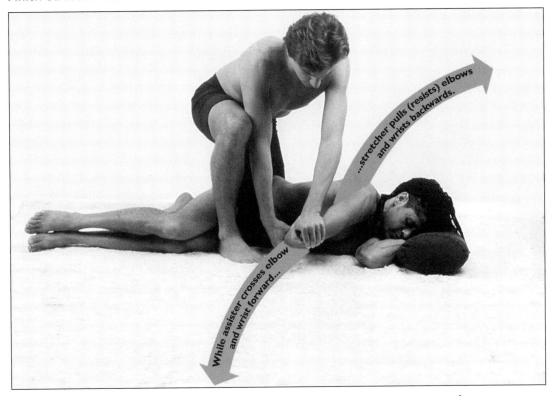

While assister crosses elbow and wrist forward...

...stretcher pulls (resists) elbows and wrists backwards.

REMEMBER: Keep resisting in position 2. Without resistance, you won't get a stretch.

Breathing

Inhale as you get into the starting position. Exhale as you move through the stretch.

Benefits

This stretch can help to improve the health of your small intestine and increase the movement of cerebrospinal fluid up your spine. Psychologically, this stretch can help you to be more creative, passionate, and romantic, and can help you to dismantle depression.

9. Assisted Back Lying Central Leg Raise (With Bent or Straight Leg) (BR)

Start Stretch Here—Position 1.

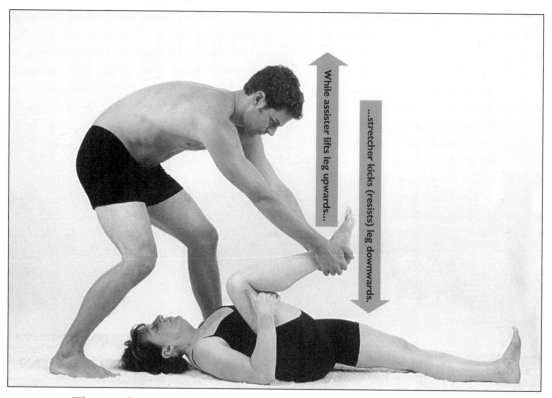

While assister lifts leg upwards...

...stretcher kicks (resists) leg downwards.

REMEMBER: The stretch occurs during the movement, not simply at the finishing position. So start resisting in position 1 and continuously resist while moving into position 2.

Getting Into This Stretch

Lie on your back and extend your legs. Bend your right knee and pull it toward your chest while keeping your left leg straight.

Adding Resistance While Stretching

Contract the muscles you are about to stretch on the back of your right leg by pulling your right heel toward your hips or by kicking your leg toward the floor as the person assisting you unbends your leg or lifts and straightens your leg toward your head. Repeat 6–10 times. Return to the starting position and change sides.

Finish Stretch Here—Position 2.

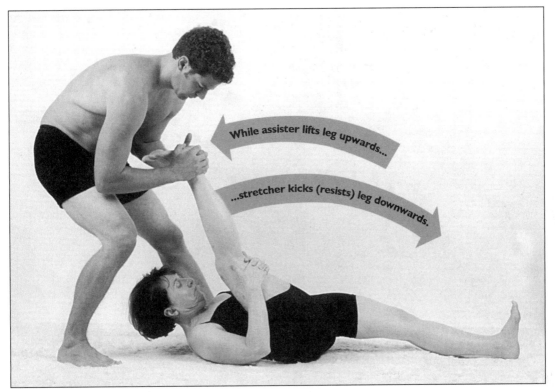

REMEMBER: Keep resisting in position 2. Without resistance, you won't get a stretch.

Breathing

Inhale as you get into the starting position. Exhale as you move through the stretch.

Benefits

This stretch can help to improve the health of your brain and central nervous system. Psychologically, this stretch can help to increase your ability to master whatever you are doing, help you to be more trusting, and can help to dismantle feelings of paranoia.

10. Assisted Hip Flexor (SE)

Start Stretch Here—Position 1.

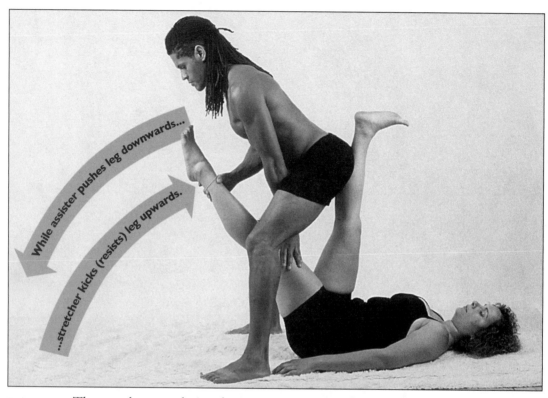

While assister pushes leg downwards...

...stretcher kicks (resists) leg upwards.

REMEMBER: The stretch occurs during the movement, not simply at the finishing position. So start resisting in position 1 and continuously resist while moving into position 2.

Getting Into This Stretch

Lie on the floor or on a bench. Extend your right leg up at a 90-degree angle with a slight bend at the knee. The person assisting you stands in front of your right leg and straddles your left leg. You can gently rest your right leg against his backside. Pull your left leg up as the person assisting you holds it by placing one hand on your ankle and the other hand just above your knee.

Adding Resistance While Stretching

Contract the muscles you are about to stretch on the front of your hip and thigh by pulling your left knee toward your chest, as the person assisting you pushes your knee toward the floor, extending your leg. Return to the starting position and repeat 6–10 times. Change sides.

Finish Stretch Here—Position 2.

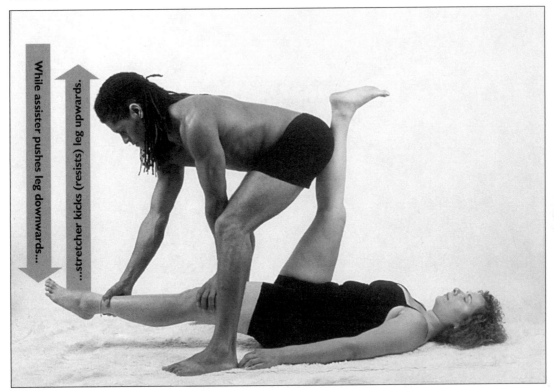

While assister pushes leg downwards...

...stretcher kicks (resists) leg upwards.

REMEMBER: Keep resisting in position 2. Without resistance, you won't get a stretch.

Breathing

Inhale as you get into the starting position. Exhale as you move through the stretch.

Benefits

This stretch can help to improve the health of your sexual organs and endocrine function, and increase your gracefulness and good looks. Psychologically, this stretch can teach you to be more caring and more accepting of yourself, and can help to dismantle your bad moods.

11. Assisted Lightning (PE)

Start Stretch Here—Position 1.

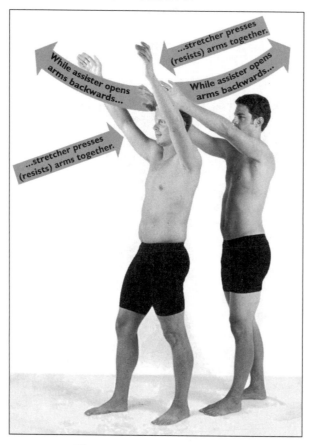

REMEMBER: The stretch occurs during the movement, not simply at the finishing position. So start resisting in position 1 and continuously resist while moving into position 2.

Getting Into This Stretch

While standing, sitting, or kneeling, raise your arms above you. The person assisting you circles your arms around and behind you.

Adding Resistance While Stretching

Contract the muscles you are about to stretch on the center front of your chest, arms, and palms, and resist the assister as he circles your arms. Return to the starting position and repeat 6–10 times.

Finish Stretch Here—Position 2.

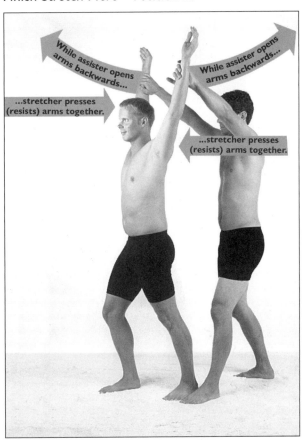

While assister opens arms backwards...

While assister opens arms backwards...

...stretcher presses (resists) arms together.

...stretcher presses (resists) arms together.

REMEMBER: Keep resisting in position 2. Without re-sistance, you won't get a stretch.

Breathing

Inhale as you get into the starting position. Exhale as you move through the stretch.

Benefits

This stretch can help to improve the health of your pericardium and increase circula-tion to your hands, feet, and genitals. Psy-chologically, this stretch can help you to be open-minded, ethical, judicious, philan-thropic, and benevolent; improve your sexual imagination; and dismantle self-defeating and self-sabotaging behaviors.

12. Assisted Thunder (SK)

Start Stretch Here—Position 1.

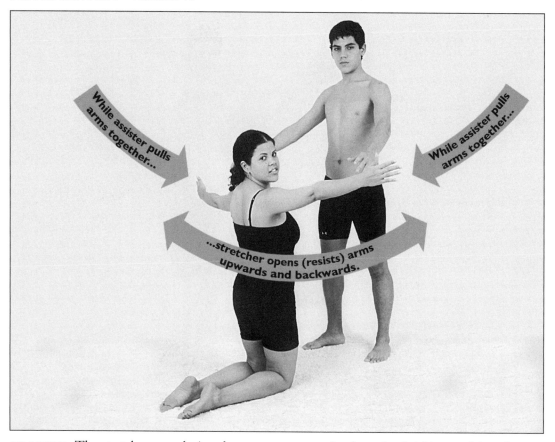

REMEMBER: The stretch occurs during the movement, not simply at the finishing position. So start resisting in position 1 and continuously resist while moving into position 2.

Getting Into This Stretch

Standing, sitting or kneeling, circle your arms above your head.

Adding Resistance While Stretching

Contract the muscles you are about to stretch on the back side of your shoulders and arms as the person assisting you brings your arms forward and downward. You are moving in a semicircular motion. Repeat 6–10 times.

Finish Stretch Here—Position 2.

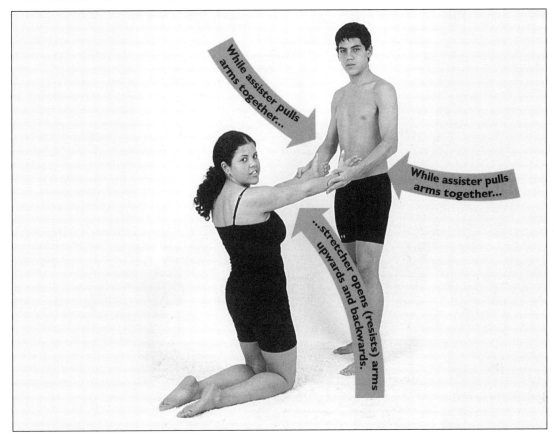

REMEMBER: Keep resisting in position 2. Without resistance, you won't get a stretch.

Breathing

Inhale as you get into the starting position. Exhale as you move through the stretch.

Benefits

This stretch can help to improve the health of your skin and external immune system. Psychologically, this stretch will teach you to better handle stress, increase your cooperativeness, help you rest, and dismantle antisocial behavior.

13. Assisted Back Lying Crossover Leg Raise (With Bent or Straight Leg) (BL)

Start Stretch Here—Position 1.

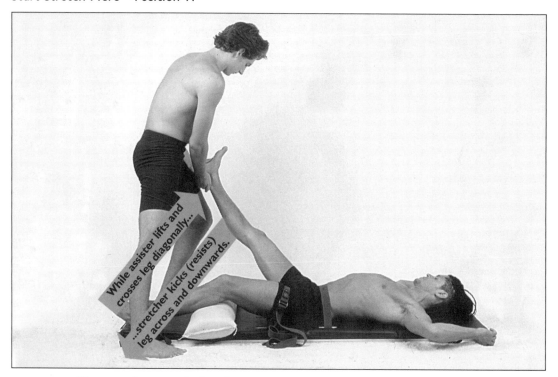

While assister lifts and crosses leg diagonally...

...stretcher kicks (resists) leg across and downwards.

REMEMBER: The stretch occurs during the movement, not simply at the finishing position. So start resisting in position 1 and continuously resist while moving into position 2.

Getting Into This Stretch

Lie on your back with your legs extended and your feet close to each other.

Adding Resistance While Stretching

Continuously contract the muscles along the back outside of the thigh that you are about to stretch by pulling your right heel toward your hips or straight leg toward the floor as the person assisting you grasps your right foot, brings your thigh across your body, and either straightens out your right leg or lifts your straight leg up toward your head. Repeat 6–10 times, then change sides.

Finish Stretch Here—Position 2.

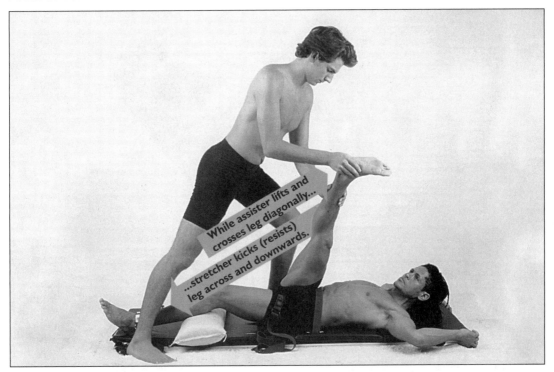

While assister lifts and crosses leg diagonally...

...stretcher kicks (resists) leg across and downwards.

REMEMBER: Keep resisting in position 2. Without resistance, you won't get a stretch.

Breathing

Inhale as you get into the starting position. Exhale as you move through the stretch.

Benefits

This stretch can help to improve the health of your bladder and your bones, improve your balance, and eliminate many back pains. Psychologically, this stretch can help to make you more hopeful and results oriented, increase your self-esteem, and dismantle narcissistic behaviors.

14. Assisted Lotus Opener (KI)

Start Stretch Here—Position 1.

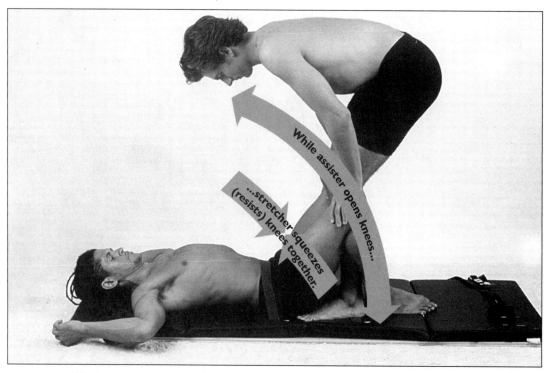

While assister opens knees...

...stretcher squeezes (resists) knees together.

REMEMBER: The stretch occurs during the movement, not simply at the finishing position. So start resisting in position 1 and continuously resist while moving into position 2.

Getting Into This Stretch

Lie on the floor with your knees together and the sides of your feet together.

Adding Resistance While Stretching

Continuously contract the muscles on the inside of your thighs that you are about to stretch by squeezing your thighs together, as the person assisting you opens your legs and pushes them toward the ground. Repeat 6–10 times.

Finish Stretch Here—Position 2.

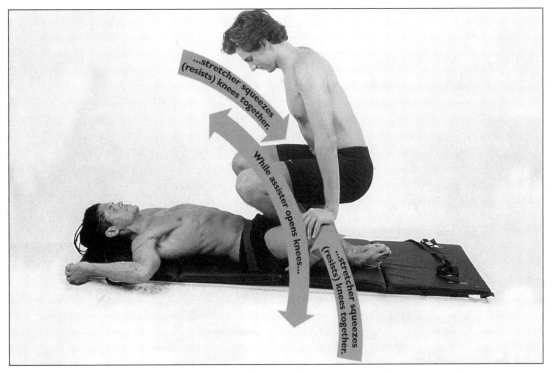

...stretcher squeezes (resists) knees together.

While assister opens knees...

...stretcher squeezes (resists) knees together.

REMEMBER: Keep resisting in position 2. Without resistance, you won't get a stretch.

Breathing

Inhale as you get into the starting position. Exhale as you move through the stretch.

Benefits

This stretch can help to improve the health of your kidneys and joints. Psychologically, this stretch may give you greater understanding and confidence, and a better sense of humor; you might become a better confidant. It also can help to dismantle "split" behaviors.

15. Assisted Back Lying Arm Change-Up (AP)

Start Stretch Here—Position 1.

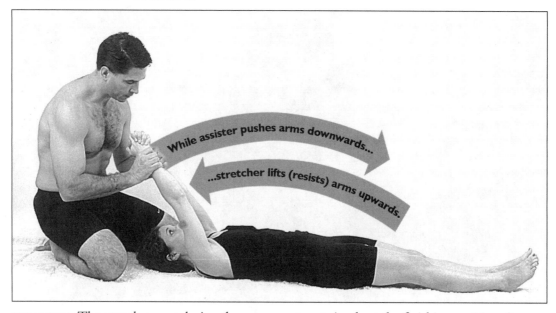

While assister pushes arms downwards...

...stretcher lifts (resists) arms upwards.

REMEMBER: The stretch occurs during the movement, not simply at the finishing position. So start resisting in position 1 and continuously resist while moving into position 2.

Getting Into This Stretch

Lie on your back and place your hands over your head, palms facing upward.

Adding Resistance While Stretching

Contract the muscles you are about to stretch on the front of your arms by pressing your hands against the person assisting you as he brings your arms down toward your waist. Return to the starting position and repeat 3 times.

Finish Stretch Here—Position 2.

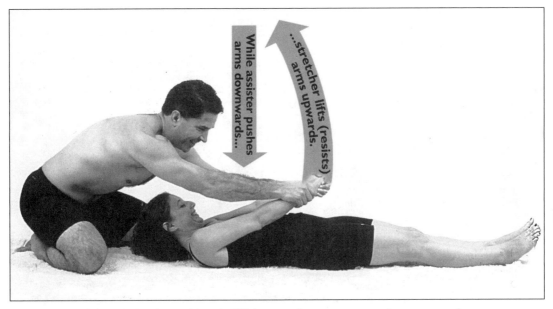

While assister pushes arms downwards...

...stretcher lifts (resists) arms upwards.

REMEMBER: Keep resisting in position 2. Without resistance, you won't get a stretch.

Breathing

Inhale as you get into the starting position. Exhale as you move through the stretch.

Benefits

This stretch can help to improve the health of your appendix and your cartilage, and help to detoxify you. Psychologically, this stretch can help you increase your capacity to change and express gratitude, help to express your individuality, and dismantle depersonalization.

16. Assisted Sunshine Arms (TH)

Start Stretch Here—Position 1.

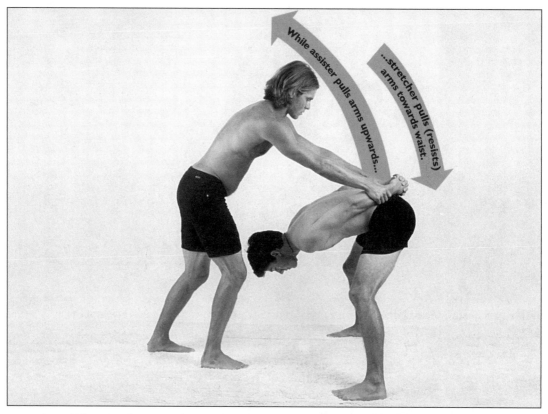

While assister pulls arms upwards...

...stretcher pulls (resists) arms towards waist.

REMEMBER: The stretch occurs during the movement, not simply at the finishing position. So start resisting in position 1 and continuously resist while moving into position 2.

Getting Into This Stretch

Stand with your legs wide apart and bend forward. Bring your arms behind your back, clasping your hands together.

Adding Resistance While Stretching

Contract the muscles you are about to stretch on the back of your shoulders and back by pulling your arms toward your hips, as the person assisting you brings your arms toward your head. Bring your head in toward your chest. Return to the starting position and repeat 6–10 times.

Finish Stretch Here—Position 2.

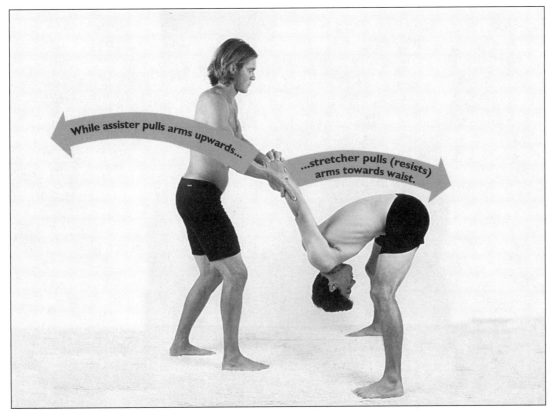

While assister pulls arms upwards...

...stretcher pulls (resists) arms towards waist.

REMEMBER: Keep resisting in position 2. Without resistance, you won't get a stretch.

Breathing

Inhale as you get into the starting position. Exhale as you move through the stretch.

Benefits

This stretch can help to improve the health of your thymus, spleen, and internal immune system. Psychologically, this stretch can increase your ability to heal and forgive, increase your hospitality skills, decrease feelings of distress, and can help to dismantle disease and brainwashing behaviors.

Chapter 13

Energy Series 4

Advanced stretch (and strength) series

1. Sphinx (GB)

Start Stretch Here—Position 1.

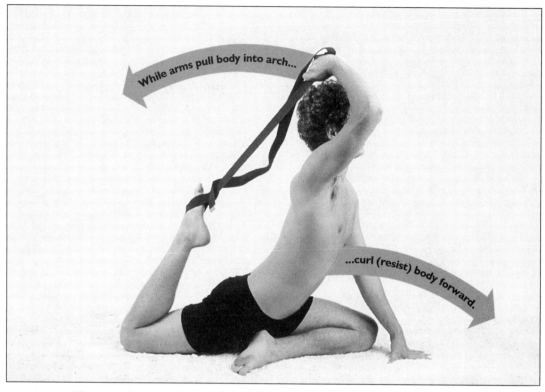

While arms pull body into arch...

...curl (resist) body forward.

REMEMBER: The stretch occurs during the movement, not simply at the finishing position. So start resisting in position 1 and continuously resist while moving into position 2.

Getting Into This Stretch

Kneel on the floor. Sit back and rest your buttocks against your heels. Bring your leg forward and cross it in front of you as you straighten your leg behind you. Your heel should rest against the front of your hip. Wrap a strap around your foot at your arch. Grasp the strap around your right foot with your hand as you bring your foot toward your head.

Adding Resistance While Stretching

Continuously contract the muscles on the side of your hip and leg by kicking your thigh and lower leg backward; also contract the muscles on the side of your torso as you resist arching backward. Return to the starting position. Repeat 6–10 times and change sides.

Finish Stretch Here—Position 2.

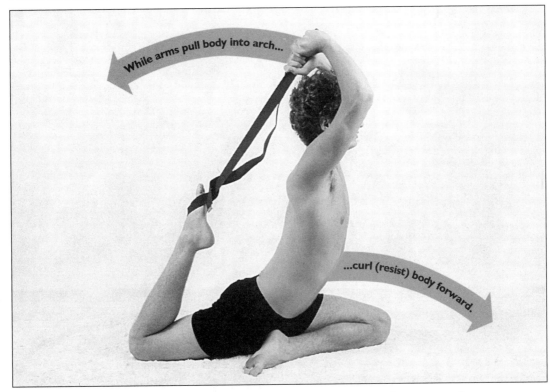

While arms pull body into arch...

...curl (resist) body forward.

REMEMBER: Keep resisting in position 2. Without resistance, you won't get a stretch.

Breathing

Inhale as you get into the starting position. Exhale as you move through the stretch.

Benefits

This stretch can help to improve the health of your gallbladder and tendons, improve fat metabolism, and increase your ability to turn from side to side. Psychologically, this stretch can help to increase your devotion, help you be certain when you are making decisions, help you to step up to the plate when the going gets tough, and can help to dismantle dependency problems.

2. Seated Lateral Bend (LV)

Start Stretch Here—Position 1.

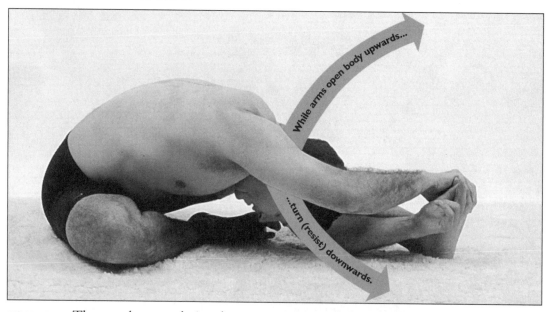

REMEMBER: The stretch occurs during the movement, not simply at the finishing position. So start resisting in position 1 and continuously resist while moving into position 2.

Getting Into This Stretch

Sit on the ground with your legs extended and spread wide apart. Bend your right knee and bring your right foot in toward your groin. Bend your torso to the left, as you grasp your left foot with both hands.

Adding Resistance While Stretching

Continuously contract the muscles on the side of your left thigh that you are about to stretch by squeezing your thighs together and resisting the turning and opening of the lateral twist. Return to the starting position. Repeat 6–10 times, then change sides.

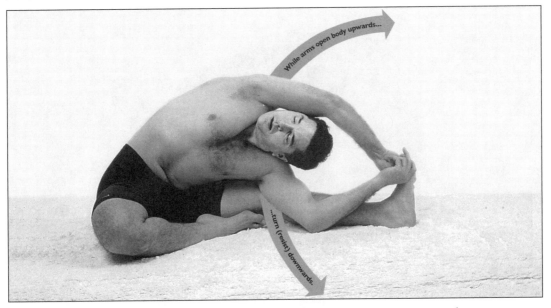

Finish Stretch Here—Position 2.

REMEMBER: Keep resisting in position 2. Without resistance, you won't get a stretch.

Breathing

Inhale as you get into the starting position. Exhale as you move through the stretch.

Benefits

This stretch can help to improve the health of your liver and tendons, detoxify you, as well as improving your overall appearance. Psychologically, this stretch can increase your awareness of what you truly desire, help you to become more helpful and less repressed, and help you to develop deeper independence while dismantling codependency.

3. Free Handstand Push-up (LU)

Start Stretch Here—Position 1.

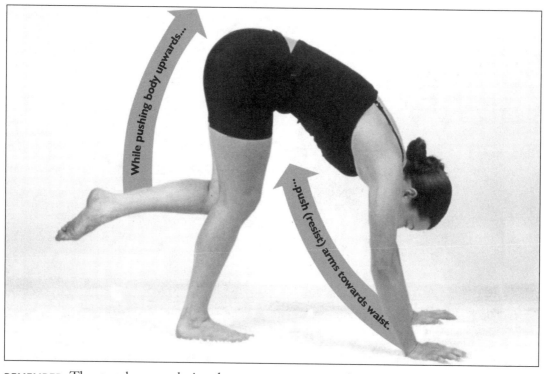

While pushing body upwards...

...push (resist) arms towards waist.

REMEMBER: The stretch occurs during the movement, not simply at the finishing position. So start resisting in position 1 and continuously resist while moving into position 2.

Getting Into This Stretch

Kneel on all fours, with your palms on the floor in front of you.

Adding Resistance While Stretching

Continuously contract the muscles you are about to stretch on the front of your chest and the inside of your arms by pressing against the floor as you kick up into a handstand. You can practice doing this stretch against a wall until you can balance in a freestanding handstand. You can also add push-ups while doing this. Return to the starting position. Repeat 6–10 times.

Breathing

Inhale as you get into the starting position. Exhale as you move through the stretch.

Benefits

This stretch can help you to improve the health of your lungs, increase the oxygen levels in your blood, improve your endurance, and increase your strength. Psychologically, the stretch can help to increase your personal power, help you to develop better boundaries, and assist you in dismantling passive-aggressive behaviors.

REMEMBER: Keep resisting in position 2. Without resistance, you won't get a stretch.

Finish Stretch Here—Position 2.

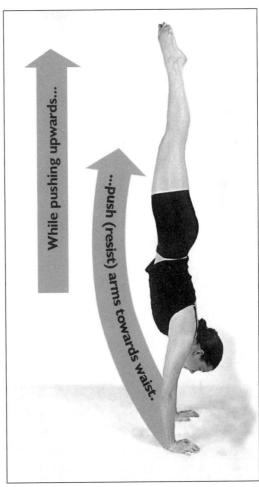

4. Inverse Kneeling Twist (LI)

Start Stretch Here—Position 1.

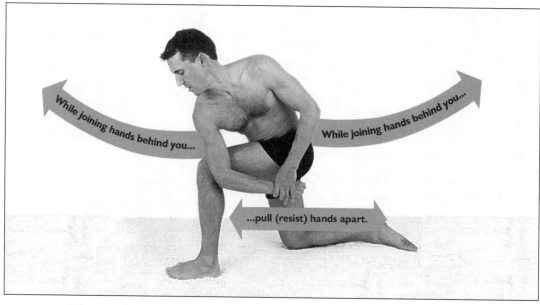

While joining hands behind you...

While joining hands behind you...

...pull (resist) hands apart.

REMEMBER: The stretch occurs during the movement, not simply at the finishing position. So start resisting in position 1 and continuously resist while moving into position 2.

Getting Into This Stretch

Kneel on the floor. Step forward onto your left foot and then turn to the left and place your right elbow on the outside of your left knee and clasp your right wrist with your left hand.

Adding Resistance While Stretching

Continuously contract the muscles on the back of your right shoulder that you are about to stretch by pressing your right elbow against your left knee, pushing your right wrist against your left hand as you push your right hand under you until you can move your left hand around your back and clasp both hands together (pull them against each other for resistance). Straighten your right leg. Release your hand clasp and return to the starting position. Repeat 6–10 times, then change sides.

Finish Stretch Here—Position 2.

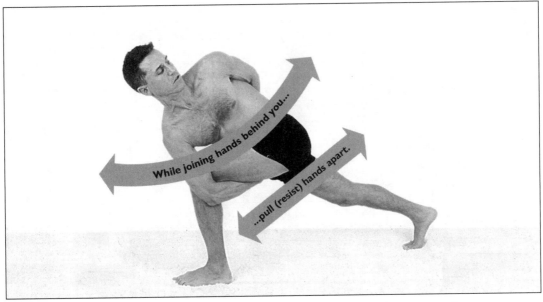

While joining hands behind you...

...pull (resist) hands apart.

REMEMBER: Keep resisting in position 2. Without resistance, you won't get a stretch.

Breathing

Inhale as you get into the starting position. Exhale as you move through the stretch.

Benefits

This stretch can help you to improve the health of your large intestine, increase venous blood flow, and improve your bowel movements. Psychologically, this stretch can help to increase your ambition, self-control, feelings of serenity, and fairness, and can help to dismantle obsessive-compulsive behaviors.

5. Backbend at the Wall (ST)

Start Stretch Here—Position 1.

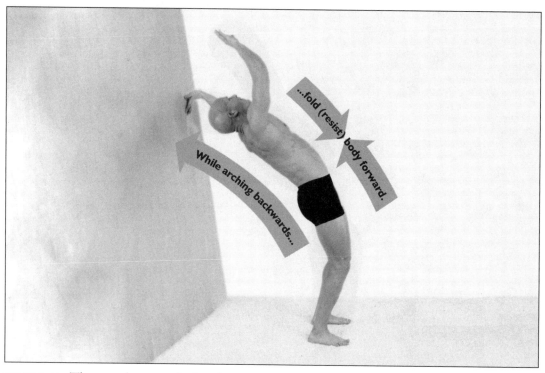

REMEMBER: The stretch occurs during the movement, not simply at the finishing position. So start resisting in position 1 and continuously resist while moving into position 2.

Getting Into This Stretch

Standing, face away from the wall, and arch backward until both hands are above your head on the wall.

Adding Resistance While Stretching

Continuously contract the muscles you are stretching on the front of your legs, torso, neck, and head by (1) kicking your lower legs forward; (2) pulling your knees up toward your chest; (3) curling your head, neck, and torso toward your waist; and (4) pressing your arms and hands against the wall as you backbend down the wall.

Finish Stretch Here—Position 2.

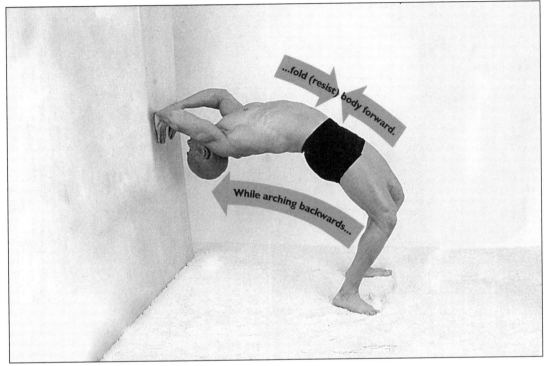

...fold (resist) body forward.

While arching backwards...

REMEMBER: Keep resisting in position 2. Without resistance, you won't get a stretch.

Breathing

Inhale as you get into the starting position. Exhale as you move through the stretch.

Benefits

This stretch can help to improve the health of your stomach and muscles, and decrease or eliminate muscular pain. Psychologically, this stretch can help to increase your sobriety, self-expression, wish fulfillment, and self-realization, and help you to develop an exceptional taste for quality and a love for work and movement. This stretch can help to dismantle addictions and eccentric behaviors.

6. Turtle (PS)

Start Stretch Here—Position 1.

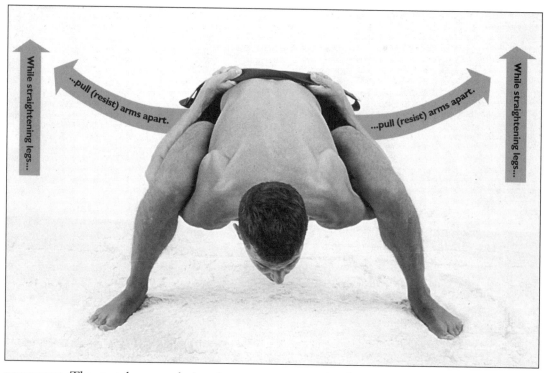

While straightening legs...

...pull (resist) arms apart.

...pull (resist) arms apart.

While straightening legs...

REMEMBER: The stretch occurs during the movement, not simply at the finishing position. So start resisting in position 1 and continuously resist while moving into position 2.

Getting Into This Stretch

Standing, open both of your legs wide. Bend over and circle your arms around your back or around your thighs to meet in the back. Clasp your hands (or use a strap to connect the hands).

Adding Resistance While Stretching

Continuously contract the muscles on the inside back of your thighs and between your shoulder blades that you are about to stretch by resisting your arms against your legs as your straighten and bend your legs. Extend your back when your knees bend, and curl your chin toward your chest as you straighten your legs. Repeat 6–10 times.

Finish Stretch Here—Position 2.

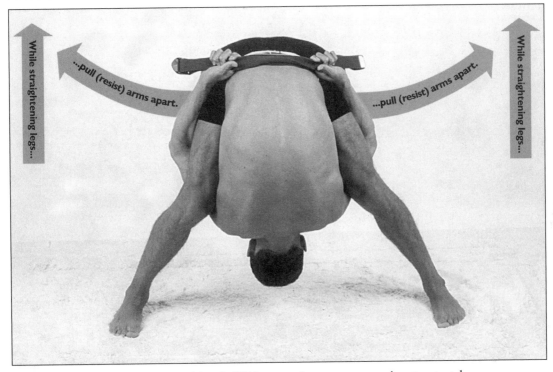

REMEMBER: Keep resisting in position 2. Without resistance, you won't get a stretch.

Breathing

Inhale as you get into the starting position. Exhale as you move through the stretch.

Benefits

This stretch can help you to improve the health of your pancreas, thus improving your digestion; increase your energy; and decrease or eliminate fascia or scar tissue damage. Psychologically, this stretch can help to increase your temperance, empathy, and communication skills, and can help you to become more playful. This stretch can assist you in dismantling indifference and move you away from feelings of martyrdom.

7. Elephant (HE)

Start Stretch Here—Position 1.

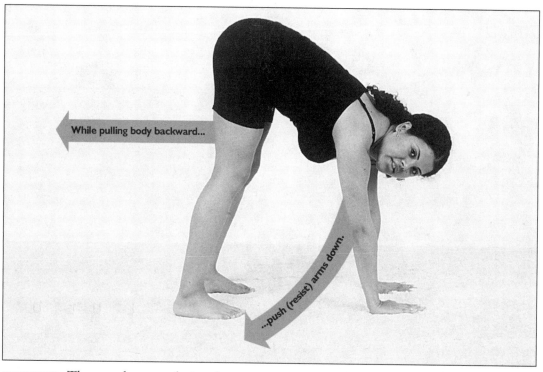

While pulling body backward...

...push (resist) arms down.

REMEMBER: The stretch occurs during the movement, not simply at the finishing position. So start resisting in position 1 and continuously resist while moving into position 2.

Getting Into This Stretch

Standing, bend at your waist. Reach forward with your hands over your head onto the floor, placing your palms in front of you.

Adding Resistance While Stretching

Continuously contract the muscles on the front of your chest and the inside of your arms into your little fingers that you are about to stretch by pulling downward toward yourself as you arch. Return to the starting position and repeat 6–10 times.

Finish Stretch Here—Position 2.

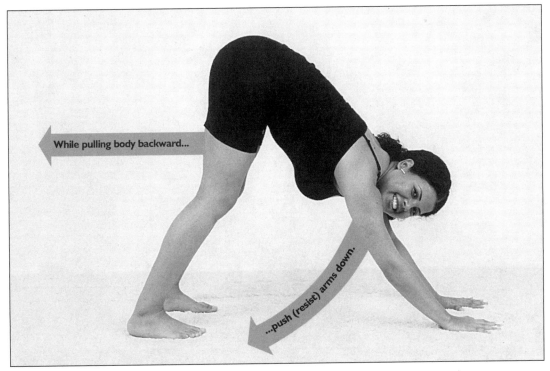

While pulling body backward...

...push (resist) arms down.

REMEMBER: Keep resisting in position 2. Without resistance, you won't get a stretch.

Breathing

Inhale as you get into the starting position. Exhale as you move through the stretch.

Benefits

This stretch can help to improve the health of your heart and increase blood flow. Psychologically, this stretch can increase your wakefulness and your ability to be unconditionally loving and joyful, improve your mediation skills, help you to know when to take action, and help you to keep momentum on projects. This stretch can also help to dismantle your sloth and avoidance.

8. Wombat (SI)

Start Stretch Here—Position 1.

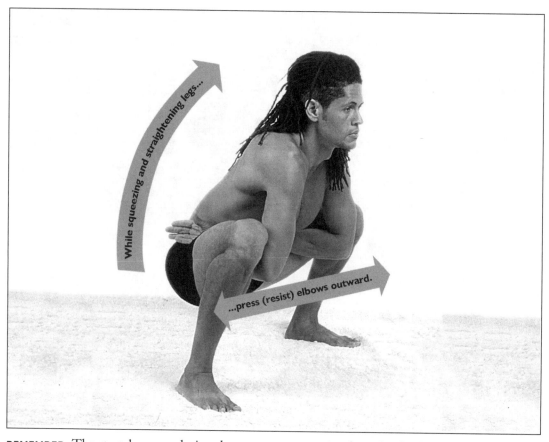

While squeezing and straightening legs...

...press (resist) elbows outward.

REMEMBER: The stretch occurs during the movement, not simply at the finishing position. So start resisting in position 1 and continuously resist while moving into position 2.

Getting Into This Stretch

From a standing position, bend both knees and move into a full squat with your buttocks resting against your calves. Spread your legs wide with your feet facing forward. Tuck your wrists into your sides as you bend forward, and place each elbow inside of your legs.

Adding Resistance While Stretching

Continuously contract the muscles on the back of your shoulders and arms that you are about to stretch as you press your elbows backward against your knees while squeezing your legs together and straightening them. Repeat this movement 6–10 times.

Finish Stretch Here—Position 2.

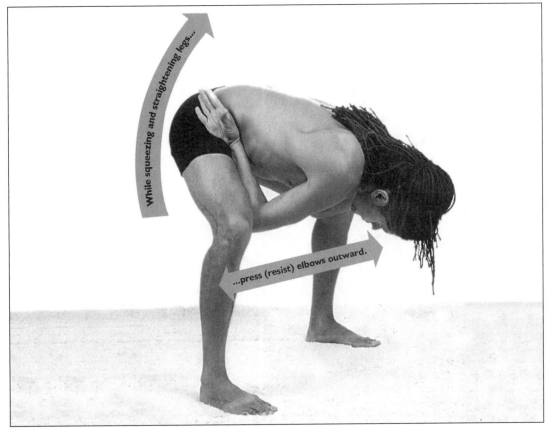

REMEMBER: Keep resisting in position 2. Without resistance, you won't get a stretch.

Breathing

Inhale as you get into the starting position. Exhale as you move through the stretch.

Benefits

This stretch can help to improve the health of your small intestine and increases cerebrospinal fluid movement up your spine. Psychologically, this stretch can help to make you more creative, passionate, and romantic, and can help to dismantle depression.

9. Inverse Seated Twist (BR)

Start Stretch Here—Position 1.

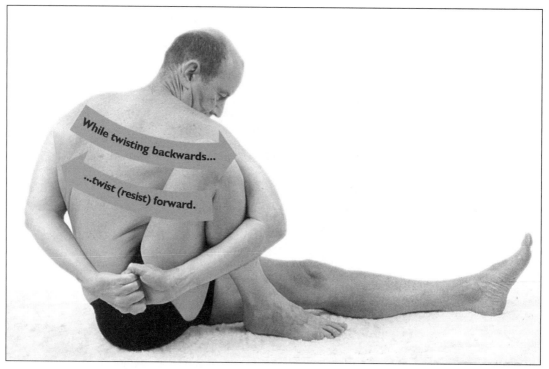

While twisting backwards...

...twist (resist) forward.

REMEMBER: The stretch occurs during the movement, not simply at the finishing position. So start resisting in position 1 and continuously resist while moving into position 2.

Getting Into This Stretch

Sit on the floor. Bend your right knee and bring your right foot next to your right thigh. Circle your arms around your right leg.

Adding Resistance While Stretching

Contract the muscles you are about to stretch on the back of your body as you resist the twisting movement in your spine and hips. Untwist and repeat 6–10 times. Change sides.

Finish Stretch Here—Position 2.

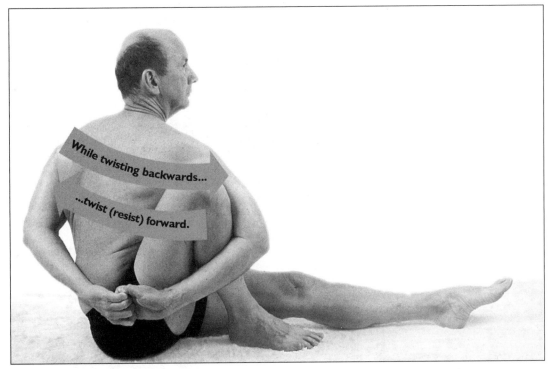

REMEMBER: Keep resisting in position 2. Without resistance, you won't get a stretch.

Breathing

Inhale as you get into the starting position. Exhale as you move through the stretch.

Benefits

This stretch can help to improve the health of your brain and central nervous system. Psychologically, this stretch can help to increase your ability to master whatever you are doing, help you to be more trusting, and can help you to dismantle feelings of paranoia.

10. Forearm Stand at Wall (SE)

Start Stretch Here—Position 1.

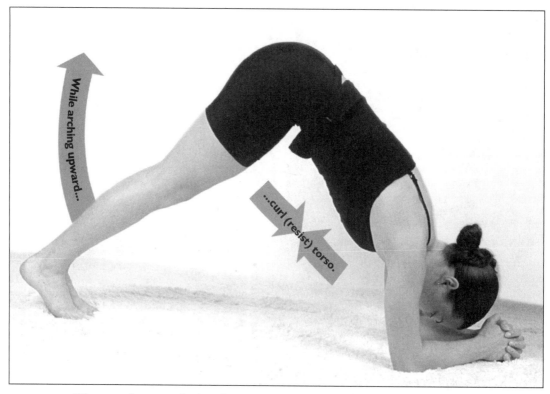

While arching upward...

...curl (resist) torso.

REMEMBER: The stretch occurs during the movement, not simply at the finishing position. So start resisting in position 1 and continuously resist while moving into position 2.

Getting Into This Stretch

Kneel on all fours. Place both forearms on the floor, palms facing downward and hands clasped, making a triangle of your hands and forearms. Lift your fanny and straighten your legs. Kick your legs up into a vertical position.

Adding Resistance While Stretching

Contract the muscles you are about to stretch on the front of your hips, thighs, and torso by contracting the muscles on the front of your body as you kick your legs up against the wall. Return to the starting position and repeat 6–10 times.

Breathing

Inhale as you get into the starting position. Exhale as you move through the stretch.

Benefits

This stretch can help to improve the health of your sexual organs and endocrine functions, increase your gracefulness, and improve your looks. Psychologically, this stretch can teach you to be more caring and more accepting of yourself, and can help to dismantle your bad moods.

REMEMBER: Keep resisting in position 2. Without resistance, you won't get a stretch.

Finish Stretch Here—Position 2.

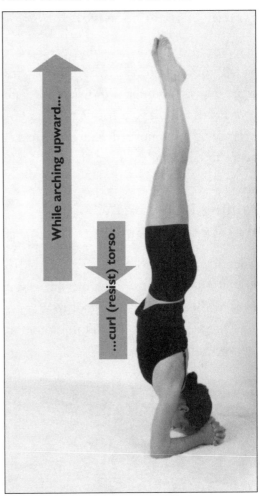

While arching upward...

...curl (resist) torso.

11. Prayer Arms Behind Your Back (PE)

Getting Into This Stretch

Standing, sitting, or kneeling, press your palms together behind your back with your fingers pointing downward. Rotate your hands toward your back until your fingers are pointing upward. Lift your pressed palms toward your shoulder blades.

Adding Resistance While Stretching

Contract the muscles you are about to stretch on the center front of your chest, arms, and palms as you attempt to unpress your hands. Return to the starting position and repeat 6–10 times.

Start Stretch Here—Position 1.

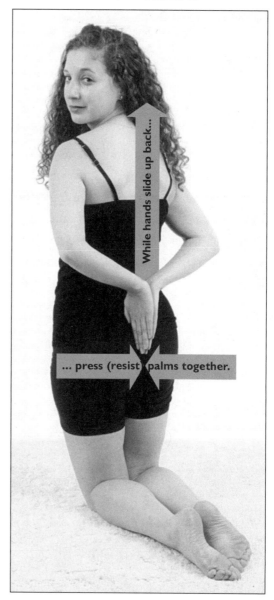

While hands slide up back...

... press (resist) palms together.

REMEMBER: The stretch occurs during the movement, not simply at the finishing position. So start resisting in position 1 and continuously resist while moving into position 2.

Breathing

Inhale as you get into the starting position. Exhale as you move through the stretch.

Benefits

This stretch can help to improve the health of your pericardium and circulation to your hands, feet, and genitals. Psychologically, this stretch can help you to be open-minded, ethical, judicious, philanthropic, and benevolent, improve your sexual imagination, and dismantle self-defeating and self-sabotaging behaviors.

Finish Stretch Here—Position 2.

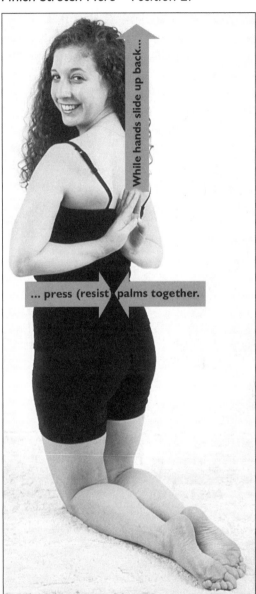

While hands slide up back...

... press (resist) palms together.

REMEMBER: Keep resisting in position 2. Without resistance, you won't get a stretch.

12. Cobra Arch (SK)

Start Stretch Here—Position 1.

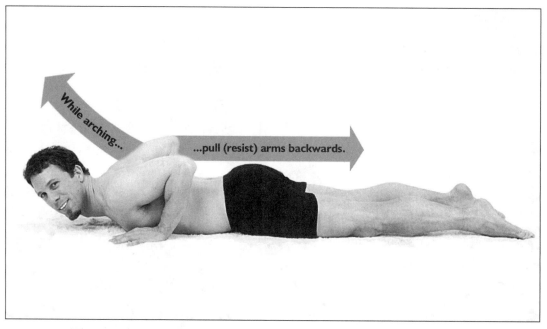

While arching...

...pull (resist) arms backwards.

REMEMBER: The stretch occurs during the movement, not simply at the finishing position. So start resisting in position 1 and continuously resist while moving into position 2.

Getting Into This Stretch

Lie prone. Place both elbows and hands parallel in front of you.

Adding Resistance While Stretching

Contract the muscles you are about to stretch on the back side of your shoulders and arms as you pull backward and push downward against the floor, raising into an arch. Lift your whole body off the ground and bend your knees, bringing your feet toward your head. Press your lower legs also against the floor. Repeat the resistance 6–10 times.

Finish Stretch Here—Position 2.

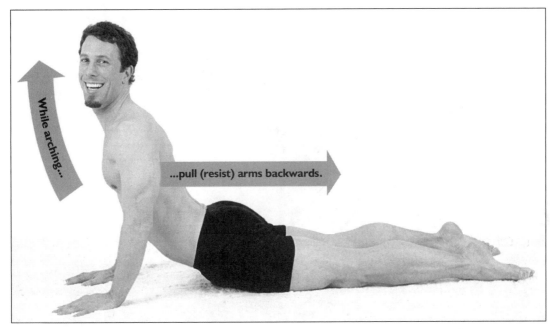

While arching...

...pull (resist) arms backwards.

REMEMBER: Keep resisting in position 2. Without resistance, you won't get a stretch.

Breathing

Inhale as you get into the starting position. Exhale as you move through the stretch.

Benefits

This stretch can help to improve the health of your skin and external immune system. Psychologically, this stretch can teach you how to better handle stress, increase your cooperativeness, and help you rest. This stretch can help to dismantle antisocial behavior.

13. One Leg Balancing (BL)

Start Stretch Here—Position 1.

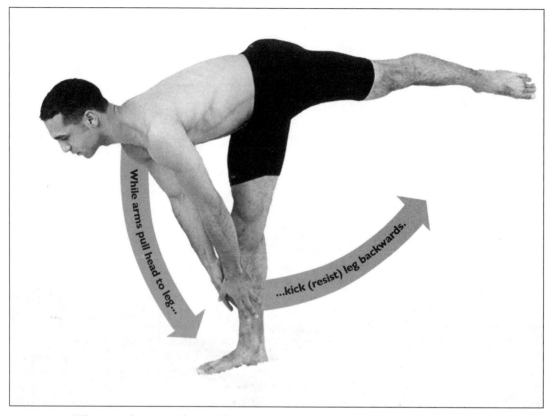

While arms pull head to leg...

...kick (resist) leg backwards.

REMEMBER: The stretch occurs during the movement, not simply at the finishing position. So start resisting in position 1 and continuously resist while moving into position 2.

Getting Into This Stretch

Standing, lift your left leg behind you until it is parallel to the floor. Bend forward and place both hands on the floor. Grasp the outside of your right ankle with your right hand, while using your other hand to help you balance.

Adding Resistance While Stretching

Continuously contract the muscles along the back outside of your thigh that you are about to stretch while you pull your torso and head toward your knee. (This has been called threading the needle.) Lower your leg and raise your torso. Repeat 6–10 times, then change sides.

Finish Stretch Here—Position 2.

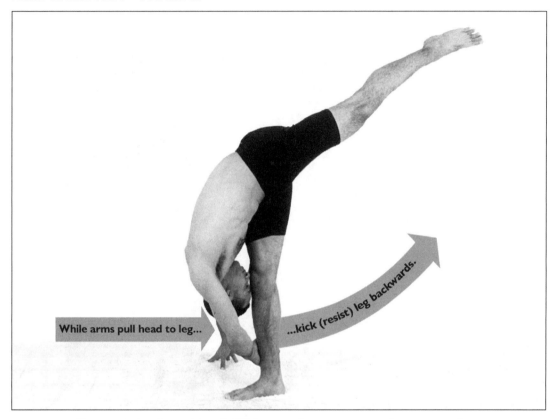

While arms pull head to leg...

...kick (resist) leg backwards.

REMEMBER: Keep resisting in position 2. Without resistance, you won't get a stretch.

Breathing

Inhale as you get into the starting position. Exhale as you move through the stretch.

Benefits

This stretch can help to improve the health of your bladder and your bones, improve your balance, and eliminate many back pains. Psychologically, this stretch can help to make you more hopeful and results oriented, increase your self-esteem, and dismantle narcissistic behaviors.

14. Rock and Roll (KI)

Start Stretch Here—Position 1.

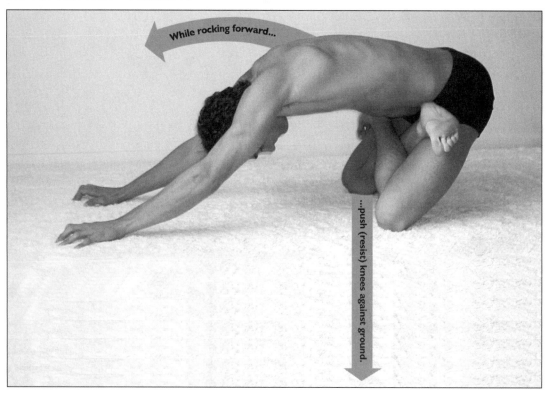

While rocking forward...

...push (resist) knees against ground.

REMEMBER: The stretch occurs during the movement, not simply at the finishing position. So start resisting in position 1 and continuously resist while moving into position 2.

Getting Into This Stretch

Sit on the floor and cross your legs into a full lotus position with each foot resting on the opposite thigh.

Adding Resistance While Stretching

Continuously contract the muscles on the inside of your thighs and front of your hips that you are about to stretch by squeezing your thighs together and pressing your knees into the floor, as you come up onto your knees and arch forward. Return to the starting position. Repeat 6–10 times.

Finish Stretch Here—Position 2.

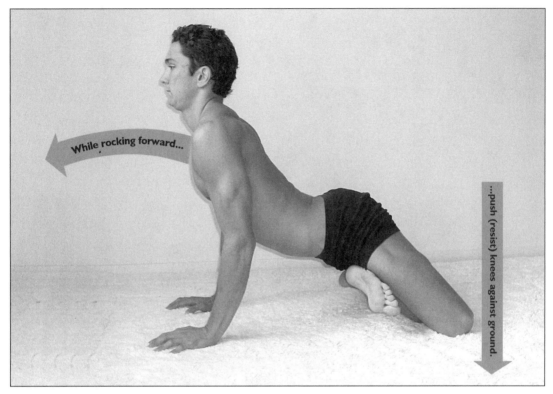

While rocking forward...

...push (resist) knees against ground.

REMEMBER: Keep resisting in position 2. Without resistance, you won't get a stretch.

Breathing

Inhale as you get into the starting position. Exhale as you move through the stretch.

Benefits

This stretch can help to improve the health of your kidneys and joints. Psychologically, this stretch will help to give you greater understanding and confidence, and a better sense of humor. This stretch can also help you to become a better confidant and dismantle "split" behaviors.

15. Full Locust at the Wall (AP)

Start Stretch Here—Position 1.

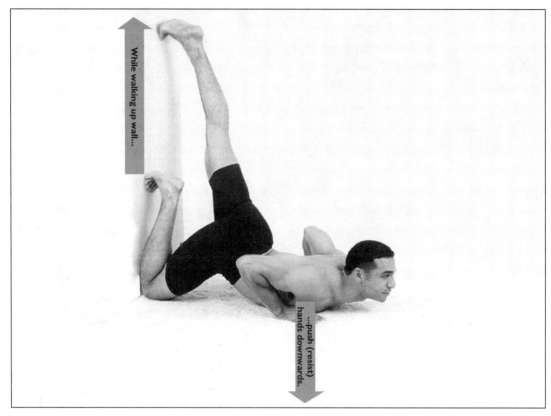

While walking up wall...

...push (resist) hands downwards.

REMEMBER: The stretch occurs during the movement, not simply at the finishing position. So start resisting in position 1 and continuously resist while moving into position 2.

Getting Into This Stretch

Kneel on the floor. Place your hands on the floor in front of you and lower your upper body into the push-up position. Point your chin forward until your throat is on the floor with your neck arched. Walk your feet up the wall until you are lifted into a full arch.

Adding Resistance While Stretching

Contract the muscles you are about to stretch on the front of your arms by pressing your hands into the floor as you lift yourself into the arch. Return to the starting position and repeat 3 times. Resist the arching maximally.

Finish Stretch Here—Position 2.

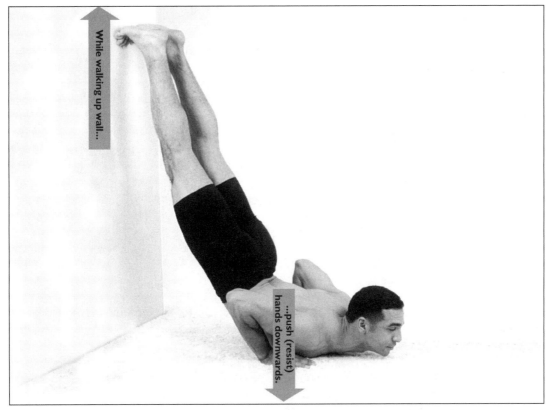

While walking up wall...

...push (resist) hands downwards.

REMEMBER: Keep resisting in position 2. Without resistance, you won't get a stretch.

Breathing

Inhale as you get into the starting position. Exhale as you move through the stretch.

Benefits

This stretch can help to improve the health of your appendix and your cartilage, and can help to detoxify your body. Psychologically, this stretch can help to increase your ability to change, express gratitude, and express your individuality, and can help to dismantle feelings of depersonalization.

16. Shoulder Bridge (TH)

Start Stretch Here—Position 1.

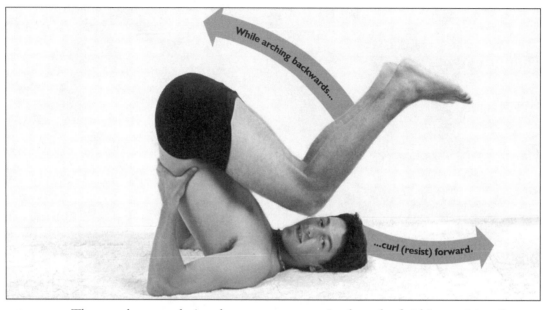

While arching backwards...

...curl (resist) forward.

REMEMBER: The stretch occurs during the movement, not simply at the finishing position. So start resisting in position 1 and continuously resist while moving into position 2.

Getting Into This Stretch

Lie on the floor on your back. Raise your hips with both feet firmly planted on the floor. Place your hands at your waist with your fingers against your back and your elbows on the floor. Curl up into a shoulder stand, bringing your feet over your head to touch the floor behind you.

Adding Resistance While Stretching

Contract the muscles you are about to stretch on the back of your shoulders and back by pushing your arms into the floor, as you lift yourself up into a shoulder stand and bring your feet over your hips and onto the ground in front of you into a backbend. Return to the starting position and repeat 6–10 times.

Finish Stretch Here—Position 2.

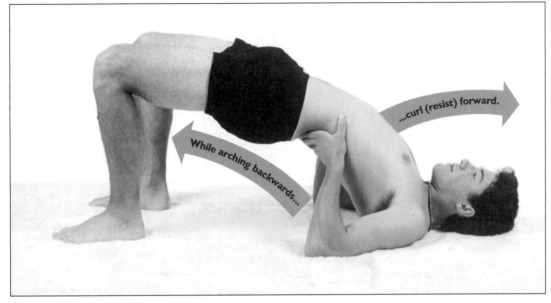

REMEMBER: Keep resisting in position 2. Without resistance, you won't get a stretch.

Breathing

Inhale as you get into the starting position. Exhale as you move through the stretch.

Benefits

This stretch can help to improve the health of your thymus, spleen, and internal immune system. Psychologically, this stretch can help to increase your ability to heal and forgive, improve your hospitality skills, decrease feelings of distress, and dismantle disease and brainwashing behaviors.

Stretching for Your Life

Part Four

Chapter 14

Maximize Your Stretching Program

Take your flexibility inventory
and learn how to move beyond

THESE FLEX SELF-TESTS can be used to increase your current level of flexibility in four different ways: physically, spiritually, emotionally, and psychologically. Use the worksheet at the end of this chapter to record those stretch numbers that describe the positive traits that you wish to develop and the negative traits that you'd like to diminish. Create an individual stretching program for yourself based on the stretches you need the most.

Young for life: Physical Fitness Flex Self-Test

It is commonly known that exercise can generally affect you physically and physiologically. But many of us have experienced that each of the different stretches can predictably affect very specific physical and physiological functions. Making any one of the muscle-meridian groups more flexible results in two things. First, you experience the positive physical features and physiological health aspects for that stretch type. At the same time, you dismantle the opposite low physiological functions.

There are three parts to this physical test.

Part I

First, take a look at the illustrations of the whole body below. Notice that different areas of the body have numbered lines. Jot down on your flex worksheet those numbers that correspond to areas of your body where you have concerns, areas where you are experiencing uncomfortable tightness, tenseness, or pain.

Create or modify your own stretching program to include those stretches that will develop the positive physiological conditions you'd like to "upgrade." Expect to see improvements in your physiological health as you improve your flexibility in each of the sixteen muscle-meridian groups. This is a great way to learn about yourself and others physiologically, and to develop in yourself those qualities you most revere in others.

Scoring: on the Flex Worksheet, record the numbers that correspond to the number of the meridian lines on your body you would like to work on.

Now try Part 2 and evaluate your physical flexibility.

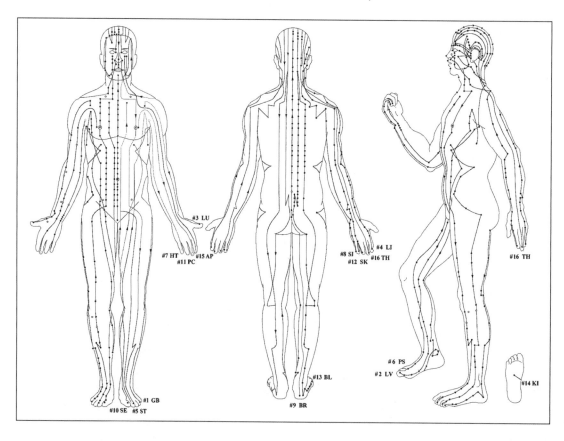

16 PHYSIOLOGICAL CONCERNS

STRETCH #	PROBLEM AREA	SYMPTOMS
1	Gallbladder	Frequent flatulence, burping, difficulty digesting fat, ligament injuries, migraine headaches, lower-back problems
2	Liver	Vision problems, hypochondriacal anxieties, tendon problems, toxicity, jaundice
3	Lungs	Inability to take a deep breath, mottled skin, weakness, lethargy, prolonged or habitual seasonal colds, lack of endurance, varicose veins, hyperextension in knees and elbows
4	Large intestine	Problems with elimination, raised and tensed shoulders, weak grip strength, venous blood flow problems, blood pressure irregularities, hypersensitive skin on top of feet, frozen shoulder, dehydration, water retention
5	Stomach	Gluttony, addiction, muscle pains or injuries, asthma, allergies, inability to sit, reading problems, digestive problems, sweet cravings, bad food combining, very irregular eating habits
6	Pancreas	Energy fluctuations, belching, heartburn, fascia hypertrophy, gum disorders, endometriosis, Epstein-Barr, autoimmune disorders, fibromyalgia, dizziness, hyperticklishness, eczema, urgency to eat every couple of hours, lack of taste, pancreas problems, acne
7	Heart	Forgetfulness, sleep disorders, excessive sweating, physical heaviness, circulation problems, heart problems
8	Small intestine	Abdominal bloating, warts, inability to gain weight, internal bleeding, anemia, gynecological disorders, lack of finger dexterity, depressed posture, wrinkles
9	Brain	Inability to remember data; right upper shoulder tension; nervousness; legs and arms feel disconnected from torso, neck, and head
10	Sexuality	Diminished sexual drive, carbohydrate cravings, overconsumption of food, weight problems, mood swings
11	Pericardium	Cold hands and/or feet, constriction of blood flow, pale skin coloring, stiffness, sleep disorders, chest pain, susceptibility to flu, runny nose
12	Skin	Skin problems, stress-related health issues, external immune problems, aversion to exercise, lymphatic flow problems, tension in back of shoulder
13	Bladder	Back problems, prostate disorders, frequent urination, bone disorders, cancer, balance problems, neurosis, hamstring and calf cramps
14	Kidney	Dark circles under the eyes, kidney stones, joint problems, arthritis, hearing difficulty, heaviness around hips, frequently feeling cold, adrenal weakness, impotence
15	Appendix	Lower right abdominal, hip, and thigh pain; appendicitis; food poisoning; bumpy complexion; difficulty completing a thought; extreme muscle tautness
16	Thymus	Internal immune disorders, swollen lymph nodes, tonsillitis, lower and upper bottom disconnect, eating disorders, general ill health

Part 2

Attempt the intermediate self-stretch series 2. Being able to comfortably get into each of the stretch positions, doing 6–10 repetitions, and resisting maximally are signs of average ranges of flexibility. Jot down on the worksheet those stretches that are difficult for you to do fully.

Part 3

Use the previous list of physiological traits to evaluate your physiological fitness. Most likely you'll discover several aspects of your physiological fitness that you'd like to improve. On the Flex Worksheet, record the numbers that correspond to the physiological conditions you want to address. Each numbered physiological condition corresponds exactly to the same numbered stretch in Part III.

Scoring: On the Flex Worksheet, jot down the numbers that correspond to the physiological conditions you'd like to work on.

Values for Life: Spiritual Fitness Flex Self-Test

It is commonly known that exercise can generally affect your energetic state. But many of us have experienced that each of the different types of stretches can predictably affect very specific spiritual traits or values. Making any of the muscle-meridian groups more flexible results in two things. First, you experience the development of a specific high spiritual virtue. At the same time, you dismantle its opposite low trait.

Use the following list of spiritual attributes to help evaluate your spiritual fitness. Most likely you'll discover several aspects of your spiritual fitness that you'd like to enhance. Check off the numbers on the Flex Worksheet that correspond to spiritual traits you want to work on. Each numbered spiritual trait corresponds exactly to the same numbered stretch in Part III.

Create or modify your own stretching program to include those stretches that develop the high spiritual values you decide you want to develop or improve in yourself. Expect to see improvements in your spiritual behavior as you increase your flexibility in each of the sixteen muscle-meridian groups.

Scoring: On the Flex Worksheet, jot down the numbers that correspond to the spiritual traits you want to work on.

In a Good Mood for Life: Emotional Fitness Flex Self-Test

It is commonly known that exercise can generally affect your emotional state. But many of us have experienced that each of the different types of stretches can predictably affect very specific emotional behaviors. Making any one of the muscle-meridian groups more flexible results in two things. First, you experience a specific high

16 SPIRITUAL FITNESS TRAITS—HIGH AND LOW

STRETCH #	HIGH PERSONALITY TRAIT	LOW PERSONALITY TRAIT
	(when being my best)	*(when not being myself)*
1	Devotional I sanctify others' lives.	Self-disloyalty I am indecisive for myself
2	Freedom I am exempt and live freely.	Codependency I am overly helpful to others.
3	Truth I have a feel for justice.	Oppression I am overly bossy.
4	Fairness I strive to be fair.	Obsessed I can't control my obsessions.
5	Belief in higher power I have a sense of a higher power.	Addiction My life centers on my addictions.
6	Peaceful I prioritize being peaceful.	Damning I am preachy and condemning.
7	Unconditional love I love faultlessly.	Sloth I am heedless and avoid intensity.
8	Equanimity I affirm others and myself.	Unaffirming I am self-denigrating and overly cautious.
9	Trust I am civil and trustworthy.	Lustful I am overly covetous.
10	Grace I give blessings and am courteous.	Empty I feel that few care, nor do I.
11	Ethical I have fair judgments.	Judgmental I sentence others unfairly.
12	Conscionable I relate to others with conscience.	Unconscionable I have no remorse.
13	Hopeful I am honest and hopeful.	Greedy I have money problems.
14	Compassionate I understand others.	Chastising I scold others about their faults.
15	Integrity I am true to my word.	Castigation I am intolerant.
16	Sisterhood-brotherhood I am forgiving.	Self-serving I am envious.

16 EMOTIONAL FITNESS TRAITS—HIGH AND LOW

STRETCH #	HIGH PERSONALITY TRAIT	LOW PERSONALITY TRAIT
	(when being my best)	(when not being myself)
1	Dependable	Undependable
	I am very devoted and loyal to others.	I lack devotion to my own life.
2	Helpful	Denial
	I take pride in helping others.	I repress my own desires.
3	Vulnerable	Unavailable
	I am deeply loving to others.	I am apathetic and removed.
4	Friendship	Depleted
	I have many friends.	I am not ambitious for myself.
5	Generous	Suggestible
	I give gifts often.	I struggle with addictions.
6	Bonding	Indifferent
	I have monogamous partners.	I am spacey and lack energy.
7	Romantic	Undiscriminating
	I am romantic in my relationships.	I do not show preferences.
8	Passionate	Abandoned
	I seek intense situations.	Others abandon me.
9	Spontaneous	Jaded
	I enjoy doing things spontaneously.	I am overly autonomous.
10	Caring	Devastated
	I take care of others always.	I am in a bad mood often.
11	Open	Closed
	I am transparent in my feelings.	I shun pleasure.
12	Community	Defensive
	I include others in what I do.	I usually feel attacked.
13	Promotional	Narcissistic
	I honestly promote everyone.	I get caught being vain.
14	Humorous	Detached
	I make others laugh.	I am overly detached.
15	Enthusiastic	Pathetic
	I am very appreciative.	I am outcast by others.
16	Hospitable	Isolated
	I welcome everyone.	I am a castle unto myself.

emotional state. At the same time, you dismantle its opposite low state.

Use the previous list of emotional merits to help evaluate your emotional fitness. Most likely you'll discover several aspects of your emotional fitness that you'd like to improve. Check the numbers on the Flex Worksheet that correspond to the emotions you wish to work on. Each numbered emo-

tion corresponds exactly to the same numbered stretch in Part III.

Create or modify your own stretching program to include the stretches that develop the positive emotions you want to upgrade. Expect to see improvements in your emotions as your flexibility increases in each of the sixteen muscle-meridian groups.

Scoring: On the Flex Worksheet, jot

16 PSYCHOLOGICAL FITNESS TRAITS—HIGH AND LOW

STRETCH #	HIGH PERSONALITY TRAIT	LOW PERSONALITY TRAIT
	(when being my best)	(when not being myself)
1	Decision making Decisive, certain, loyal, dependable, courageous	Dependency Indecisive, guilty, cowardly, secretive, demeaning
2	Freedom Liberated, unrepressed, free-spirited, humble, proud, helpful, giving, independent	Codependency Overly helpful, stuck, denying, irritable, frustrated
3	Leadership Truth seeking, discerning, powerful, strong, protective, vulnerable	Passive-aggressive Manipulative, tyrannical, autocratic, grieving, powerless, oppressive
4	Ambition Completing, perfecting, idealistic, fair, principled, serene, resolved	Obsessive-compulsive Hypercritical, controlling, procrastinating, stoic, manic
5	Sobriety Self-expressive, self-educated, work identifying, nonaddictive, sympathetic, potential promoting, tasteful, optimistic	Addiction Addictive, eccentric, digressive, vague, loose associations, overly frank
6	Peaceful Communicative, empathetic, healthy routines, aware of connections, synchronicity	Martyrdom Self-sacrificing, indifferent, moralizing, prudish, preachy, complaining, listless
7	Unconditional love Right acting, unifying, mediating, animated, solid, cheerful, imaginative, sincere	Avoidant Lazy, inert, heavy, neglectful, fiery outbursts, forgetful

16 PSYCHOLOGICAL FITNESS TRAITS—HIGH AND LOW (cont.)

STRETCH #	HIGH PERSONALITY TRAIT	LOW PERSONALITY TRAIT
	(when being my best)	(when not being myself)
8	Creativity Passionate, equable, classy, self-affirming, aesthetic, beautifying, cultured, expressive, elegant, fulfillment seeking	Depression Hysterical, self-abandoning, melancholic, self-incriminating, discouraged
9	Trust Masterful, civil, knowledgeable, cultivated, aristocratic, problem solving, happy, genteel, mantra generating, heroic	Paranoid Distrustful, delusional, betraying, lustful, nervous, covetous, rude
10	Self-worth Caring, graceful, sexual, respectful, good-looking, captivating, alluring, mood affecting, spontaneous, desirable	Moody Biased, bad habits, presumptuous, moody, empty, borderline, erratic, morbid, unstable
11	Good judgment Ethical, open, prudent, undisguised, karmic perceptive, philanthropic, transparent, validating, straightforward	Masochistic Self-defeating, oblivious, stiff, closed, sentencing, implacable
12	Athletic Risk taking, lucky, stylish, restful, vigorous, revering, community connected	Sadistic Stressed, duplicitous, antisocial, violent, mean, intimidating, lying, obnoxious, loud, enslaving
13	Promotional Honest, hopeful, successful, balanced, fiscally astute, motivating, cooperative, performing	Narcissistic Vain, anxious about failure, deceitful, narcissistic, aggrandizing, exploitative
14	Philosophical Observant, wizardly, original, innovative, enlightened, meditative, ruminating, meaning seeking, humorous	Schizoid Split, fearful, withdrawn, rejecting, greedy, regressive, retreating
15	Changeable Individualistic, integrity, enthusiastic, centered, calm	Depersonalized Out of body, anarchist, frantic, officious, toxic
16	Good health habits Healthy diet and exercise, healing, forgiving, hospitable, myth personifying	Brainwashing Troubled, diseased, angst ridden, demanding, eating disorders, destruction of property

down the numbers that correspond to the emotional traits you want to work on.

Clear-minded for Life: Psychological Fitness Flex Self-Test

It is commonly known that exercise can generally affect your mental state. But many of the people performing these stretches have experienced that each of the stretches can predictably affect very specific psychological character traits. Making any one of the muscle-meridian groups more flexible results in two things. First, you experience the high side of one of the personality type's mental states. At the same time, you dismantle its opposite low side.

Use the previous list of personality traits to help evaluate your psychological fitness. Most likely you'll discover several aspects of your mental fitness that you'd like to upgrade. Check off the numbers on the Flex Worksheet that correspond to the psychological traits you want to address. Each numbered behavioral trait corresponds exactly to the same numbered stretch in Part III.

Create or modify your own stretching program to include those stretches that develop the high personality traits you want to upgrade in yourself. Expect to see improvements in your psychological well-being as you improve your flexibility in each one of the sixteen muscle-meridian groups.

This is a great way to learn about yourself and others psychologically and to develop in yourself those qualities you most revere in others.

Scoring: On the Flex Worksheet, jot down the numbers that correspond to the psychological traits you want to work on.

FLEX WORKSHEET

STRETCH #	PHYSICAL	SPIRITUAL	EMOTIONAL	MENTAL
1				
2				
3				
4				
5				
6				
7				
8				
9				
10				
11				
12				
13				
14				
15				
16				

Chapter 15

Preventing Injury When Stretching

Bend, but do not break: overstretching

ALL RIGHT! We've covered the fundamentals of resistance stretching and now you know that you can become more flexible than you've dared to imagine. But I don't want you just to *try* stretching; I want you to *love it.* Even though you will have many unexpected successes right off the bat, you also will most likely make tons of mistakes in the beginning. Everyone does—that's how we learn. But don't get discouraged or stopped in your tracks. It has always been my absolute first priority to avoid injury.

I want you to become more flexible. You want you to become more flexible. But turning yourself into a piece of limp spaghetti is not the way to do it. Keep the following key things in mind in order to avoid overstretching.

Let Your Body Be the Authority

Your body would love you to become more conversant with it. Decide what stretch or strengthening move you want to do and then absolutely let your body lead you. Learn when you're making the mistake of thinking or feeling you know how to move better than your body does. It takes time to learn how to listen to your body. The more you yield to your body, the faster you get results. You should always feel good and comfortable when you stretch. You will expose tenseness you never knew you had, but you must learn to differentiate this old tenseness from getting yourself into awkward positions that strain you. Talk to other experienced stretchers. Ask them what they feel in particular stretches. They're a great storehouse of knowledge for you. If what they experience is radically different from what you experience, reconsider what you're doing and ask for more help.

Sustain Your Resistance

Keep resisting regardless of whether you perceive the stretch as easy or light. You must resist the entire time you are elongating a muscle. If you don't do this, your muscles, joints, or other soft tissues can be damaged. Don't risk it. Remember, if you don't feel as if you can maximally resist at any point during the stretch, then you are overstretching. It's that simple.

Stay Strong

Test your muscles to see if they are as strong as they need to be *before* you stretch. You can strength-train any muscle by simply reversing the direction of the movement you take to stretch the muscle. So if you are stretching your biceps, you start with your muscle being short and move to a position where it is long, while resisting. To strengthen, simply start with your muscle being long and move to a position where it is short, while resisting. Remember, 6–10 reps for strength training are necessary to increase the strength of your muscles—the same as with stretching. Again, your muscle will indicate whether it wants to strengthen or stretch. If you try stretching and it feels uncomfortable, then try strengthening those muscles and see if you like the way that feels. You contract your muscles when stretching, so if they are not strong enough to contract maximally throughout the stretch, then you must strength-train them first. Strengthen the muscles first, if you need to, and then stretch them. *Be safe.*

Check Your Intensity Through Breathing

Breathe any way you need to to regulate your tension and relaxation levels when you stretch. If your breathing starts to go wacko, it's best to back off and lessen your intensity. That is, change the direction of the movement or decrease your range of motion, speed, force, and duration. If you are not aware of your tenseness, then you cannot relax. When you pay attention to your tenseness and tightness, you discover that your breathing naturally changes and the result is that you relax.

Keep Your Mind in Your Head

If you cannot stay conscious and focused on what you are experiencing when stretching, then you've gone too far. If your mind wanders (you disengage) when stretching, it's comparable to sitting in a fast-moving car without a driver—very bad news. At any time during the stretch you should be able to converse with another person about what you are aware of and experiencing. If you can't, then change your action by slowing down, changing position, decreasing your force, breathing more naturally, and reducing your resistance—and have a fun and safe time instead.

Keep the Lines of Communication Flowing

When someone assists you, it is imperative that you maintain responsibility for yourself and not allow her to overstretch you. An overzealous partner can hurt you if you're not verbalizing and she's not listening. Make sure you can maximally resist, regardless of the range she takes you into. Keep an ongoing dialogue with the assister. Tell her what you feel. Have her tell you what she feels is happening to you. Help guide her into what feels good for you. When you've

had enough, agree in advance that "okay" means that you're done. (Remember to thank her.)

Stay in Your Body

You are much more likely to overstretch by staying in a stretch for a long time than by repeating a stretch. If your breathing becomes too shallow or overly dramatic, it is a sure sign you are out of bounds. You should be able to feel your body resist whether you are moving or not. When you begin to lose the feeling of your body, stop what you are doing and return to a safer way to stretch.

Balancing Asymmetries: Keeping Yourself in Line

Becoming more symmetrical happens naturally from stretching. But at some point, you need to address chronic and deep soft tissue differences that are causing imbalances in your posture and movements. Here are some things to consider.

Removing asymmetrical compensations

No one is perfectly symmetrical, but some people are more symmetrical than others. Becoming too asymmetrical places very specific stresses on your body that can eventually stop you from engaging in the physical activities that you enjoy so much. Basically, if a muscle is habitually tight on one side of your body, the balancing muscle group is tight on your other side. So if your left quad is tight, then your left hamstring is tight too. Likewise, if your left thigh is habitually externally rotated, then your right thigh compensates and habitually internally rotates. The two sides of your body generally compensate in this way. Though it is easier said than done, you can systematically remove excessive asymmetries like these by paying attention to the differences that you discover while stretching and removing blatant differences by doing repeats of those needed stretches. You might not be able at first to identify these compensations, so this is another area where other people who stretch can give you feedback on how the two sides of a body are different. You'll love how good it will make you feel.

Counterbalancing muscle groups

Each muscle group has a balancing muscle group on the opposite side of your body. For example, your quads and hamstrings, generally speaking, are balancing muscle groups for each other. Your biceps and triceps in your arms are also balancing muscle groups. Each of these groups is directly across from one other through the center of your body. But the muscle groups that are perpendicular to these two balancing muscle groups are called the counterbalancing muscle groups. These counterbalancing muscle groups keep your body in balance. For example, while

your quads and hamstrings are balancing muscle groups, your central adductors and abductors (inner and outer thigh muscles) counterbalance them and are thus called the counterbalancing muscle groups to your quads and hamstrings.

If a target group of muscles in your body is habitually tight, you may be able to stretch just those muscles and the tension will leave. When this doesn't work, the balancing muscle group needs to be stretched first before the habitual tension in your target muscle group loosens. But if stretching the target muscles or stretching the balancing muscle group doesn't result in your target muscle group relaxing, then stretch the counterbalancing muscle groups and see if that does the trick.

Let's say you try to bend over to touch the ground in front of you. If the muscles on the back of your legs (your hamstrings) are flexible, then you probably assume you can touch the ground with no difficulty and get a great stretch of these muscles in the process. But what if you can't, and why not?

You probably think the reason you can't bend forward as much as you want to is that your hamstrings are too short. But this is not always true! If you are not successful in stretching a certain set of muscles, then the muscles on the opposite side of your body need to be stretched first so that they can contract and pull you into the stretch. For example, when you want to bend forward to stretch your hamstrings, if the muscles on the front of your thighs (your quads) are too inflexible, and thus cannot contract and shorten enough, then they cannot bend you forward enough to stretch your hamstrings. But if they are sufficiently flexible, then you can bend forward and stretch your hamstrings. It's strange but true.

Let's try another example. You are trying to stretch the muscles on the front of your thighs (your quads) by folding your lower leg up toward the back of your hips. The quads will be able to stretch if the muscles on the back of your thighs (your hamstrings) are able to contract and shorten enough and bring your heels toward your hips. But if they

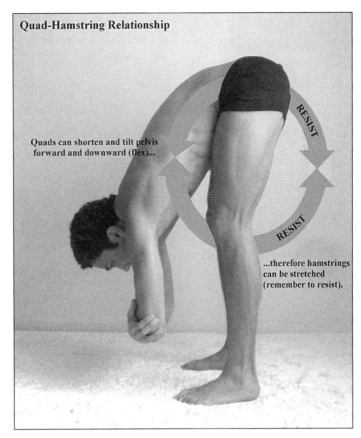

Quad-Hamstring Relationship

Quads can shorten and tilt pelvis forward and downward (flex)...

RESIST

RESIST

...therefore hamstrings can be stretched (remember to resist).

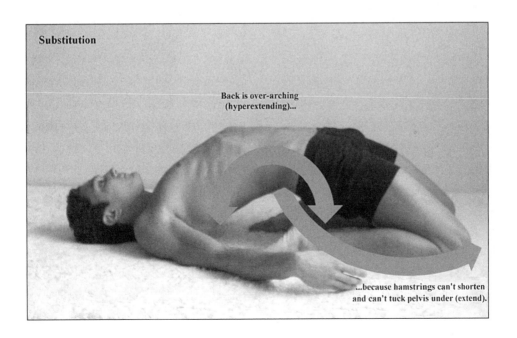

Substitution

Back is over-arching (hyperextending)...

...because hamstrings can't shorten and can't tuck pelvis under (extend).

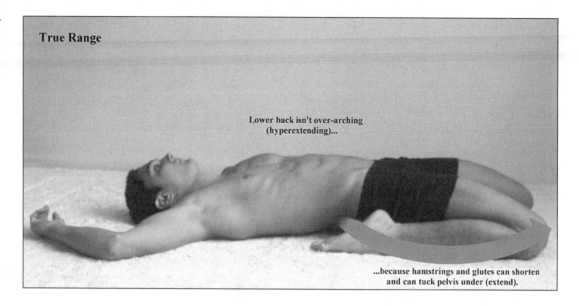

True Range

Lower back isn't over-arching (hyperextending)...

...because hamstrings and glutes can shorten and can tuck pelvis under (extend).

are not, then you will need to stretch your hamstrings first, so that they are capable of shortening and contracting enough to pull your heels toward your glutes, before you can stretch your quads.

Injuries have resulted in you being crooked

When there is too great a difference in range of motion or strength between the two sides of your body, I recommend this strategy to address your imbalance or asymmetry. Even one injured muscle can throw the rest of you into a twisted mess. Finding that muscle is the first step.

Carefully test each of the eight muscle groups in both your lower and upper body by stretching and strengthening each muscle until you find perhaps the one muscle or muscle group that is causing havoc everywhere else.

You want to stretch that one target muscle, but you find that it fatigues very quickly. So stretch and/or strengthen it, then give it a rest break and move on to the other muscles. Keep coming back to this renegade muscle until you can feel that the muscle simply cannot work anymore. You might find that you end up stretching and strengthening it five or six times more than all the other muscles in that leg or arm or your torso. You will notice immediate results if you use this strategy. Come back to it the next time you stretch and persevere until that rascal is in line with all the rest. Congratulations on your efforts. You'll love how the rest of you unravels as you remove the snag.

Keep both sides satisfied

Every energy series is composed of sixteen stretches for sixteen different muscle groups. Each stretch is followed by another stretch that works the balancing muscles (those on the opposite side of your body). Examples are your quads and hamstrings, or your abductors and abductors of your thighs. In Western anatomy, these are called agonist and antagonist muscle groups, but I call them balancing muscle groups.

Don't leave yourself hanging

Whenever you stretch in one direction, the next position should move in the opposite direction. It's simple in principle, and we all seem to do this naturally when we're paying attention to what our bodies want to do. For example, if you do a stretch that bends your body backward, then for the next stretch, bend your body forward; if your arms open sideways, then on the next stretch, close them.

You wouldn't stretch your right leg and then neglect to stretch your left leg, would you? That would really leave you hanging! By the end of your stretch routine, your whole body should feel that every muscle has been given its fair shake, so to speak.

Go into it hips first

Always stretch the muscles in your hips and legs first, then the same muscles in your arms. Your arms "sit" on top of your legs, so leg stretches always precede arm stretches. Some people are more leg dominant and some are more arm dominant. But regardless of dominance, everyone must stretch

the legs first (unless, of course, some emergency demands that you "fix" the arms first).

Balance in three directions

Your body balances itself not only from right to left and from top to bottom, but also diagonally. For example, if the front of your thigh is inflexible, then the back of your thigh will also be inflexible. In addition, if your left thigh is overly rotated outward, your right thigh will overly rotate inward, and your left arm will then overly rotate inward and your right arm will overly rotate outward—relatively speaking. There are many complex examples of this substitutional dynamic. (Check out our Web page, www.MeredianStretching.com, if your technical curiosity demands that you learn more about these sometimes complicated compensations.)

If this seems a little complex, simply start by making all the stretches pretty much the same on both sides of the body. Then you'll probably want to talk to someone who has stretched for a while. A veteran stretcher or trainer can give you some very helpful recommendations about what stretches to do to balance yourself in all directions.

Don't let the boat list

Many sports are asymmetrical—tennis and golf for example. Try—to the best of your abilities—to keep the ranges of motion and strength equal enough so that you don't become too structurally imbalanced. One-sided sports require that you become especially attentive to imbalances. Again, a knowledgeable stretcher can help you analyze your asymmetries and keep your strength and flexibility within an acceptable range of deviation.

Dim sum

Variety in activity helps to clue you in on asymmetries in your body and movements. Use significant aerobic and strength training to fill out your physical development. Cross training or simply being involved in many different movement activities will give you the variety that your body likes.

Understretching

There are more people who stretch too little than who stretch too much. But it is important to acknowledge that if you involve yourself in any physical activity, your flexibility single-handedly determines how you are going to be able to move (and keep moving, for that matter). There are also many people who do not do justice to themselves in the way they stretch. They usually have not heard about resistance stretching and characteristically don't expect much from their little warm-up stretches. There are even a good number of people who stretch daily—and enjoy the benefits they derive from their stretch routines—but are

getting very little bang for their buck, so to speak. Moderate practice of resistance stretching has been consistently shown to equal and even surpass many years of other kinds of stretching or yoga. You've got an incredible advantage and secret weapon in resistance stretching. Don't settle for anything less than what you think stretching should bring you.

A Good Kind of Sore

Soreness is a double-edged sword. When you experience a good feeling of soreness, you know that you've had a really good workout. But if you feel badly sore, you know you overdid it, or did something wrong that needs to be identified and corrected. How do you increase your chances of having good soreness and also dramatically reduce the time it takes to recover?

A lot of different things play an important role in your body's resiliency and effectiveness at reducing or eliminating soreness and speeding your recovery. Just the right amount of training, great food and hydration, and sufficient vitamin and mineral supplementation all positively affect your recovery. Great relationships, fulfilling work, positive psychological attributes, and satisfied desires lift your body's efforts to right itself through stretching and exercise.

As you stretch and work out, take a proactive approach to minimizing your poststretching soreness and maximizing recovery.

Factors That Impact Your Degree of Soreness

With resistance stretching, your degree of soreness depends on the following.

Your physical fitness level

Your aerobic health directly correlates to your ability to remove the waste products that are generated when you work out. Aerobic exercise, both before and after stretching, greatly reduces, and even eliminates, soreness.

Your skill level

Most regular stretchers find that they are mildly sore for the first several weeks (particularly if they are not accustomed to exercising daily). But I've never known anyone who didn't get over this in time. The more your body acclimates itself to resistance and to new stretch movements, the more your soreness will become a thing of the past.

The frequency of your practice

A lot of people start stretching three times per week. This quickly turns into stretching at least a little nearly every day. People who are very physically active discover that they like to stretch immediately following their aerobic exercise, as well as in the morning when they first get up. The more frequently you stretch, the faster you break through

any residual feelings of stiffness or soreness that beginners experience. You begin to feel as if you inhabit a very young person's body.

The intensity of your practice

The intensity of your stretching routine or workout, including your speed and use of maximum resistance, can dramatically affect your level of soreness. Characteristically, the greater the intensity, the greater the soreness, but only when you are first learning to stretch. Mature athletes actually experience less soreness when they pump up their resistance levels. They've discovered that maximum exertion actually turns on their immune systems, rapidly removing almost all the soreness that you might expect to experience from an intense workout.

The duration of your practice

Beginners usually stretch for fifteen to thirty minutes. But people who practice daily for greater lengths of time—forty-five minutes to two or more hours—experience about the same amount of soreness or less. Increasing the time you spend stretching seems to decrease the soreness, the opposite of what you might expect.

The time of day you practice

Early morning between 5:30 and 8:00 A.M. is the best time to stretch. Yes, you also need to stretch after your afternoon workout, but when you stretch in the morning, you change the way you are all day. Stretching only at night is like fixing up your house to sell it when you've spent years living in it unfinished, meaning that if you change the way you are going to be by stretching in the morning, then the rest of your day is guaranteed to be better and different than it usually is. But at night you are undoing and unwinding after what has already happened. That's good too, but why not have less to undo?

Some people find that stretching before they go to bed facilitates a good night's sleep and can help with insomnia, while others report greater soreness from late evening stretches.

Your physiological health

Your internal health, as it is reflected in your tissue health, significantly affects your ability to handle stretching or any kind of physical stress you place on yourself. Improve your tissue's physiological health by eating nutrient-rich, organic food, and your soreness evaporates.

Your psychological fitness

Stretching dramatically improves your psychological health. As your particular problems improve, you can expect a parallel upgrade of your body.

Your sophistication in breathing

Natural, great ways to breathe determine your tension and relaxation levels. Learning how to breathe well is essential to relaxing and enjoying your stretch, which in turn diminishes soreness.

Your pace, level of difficulty, and transitioning

Many first-time stretchers have a reach that exceeds their grasp . . . literally. They try to force their bodies into stretches they're simply not ready for. Although it's great to set goals for yourself in stretching, you need to ease into the experience. The stretches in this book are organized into beginning, intermediate, assisted and advanced levels. Start out at the beginner's level and master the basics first. Not only will you protect yourself from injury and soreness, but you also will learn more about the mechanics of each stretch. Don't become cavalier about what you are doing.

Getting into and coming out of a stretch are two very critical moments, requiring control and concentration. Moving too quickly or erratically in and out of a stretch can result in soreness and injury.

Make It Last

So, you've just finished a fantastic stretch. You're feeling wonderfully invigorated and relaxed at the same time. But the stretching experience doesn't end when you roll up the mat and hit the sauna and shower. You continue to process your stretch throughout the day, both physically and mentally. Here are few tips for making your stretching experience the best it can be each and every time.

Stretch

After a day of intense stretching, the next morning I can hardly wait to stretch, even if it's just for fifteen minutes. That's all it takes usually to put me right back on top of the great feelings I had the previous day.

Mashing: the resistance stretcher's massage

There are many different massage techniques. Pick the one that works for you. There are energetic and laying-on-of-hands healing massages, which are invigorating and relaxing at the same time. I like it when people literally walk on my back and the front of my legs and arms (we stretchers call this "mashing"). Deep weight kneading and rigorous shaking really relax me and help to increase my circulation, lymph flow and, thus, recovery. Massages can reduce your recovery time by half by increasing blood flow and removing waste products. Vigorous massage is suggested for athletes.

Eat right and drink spring water

Hydrating your body with quality drinking water, eating certified organic foods, and supplementing your food with whole-food vitamins and minerals enhance your body's energy and are essential to maintaining and sustaining your flexibility gains. Spring water is especially effective at ridding the body of harmful toxins.

You need variety—cross-train

Flexibility and aerobic and strength training all depend on one another. One without the others impedes progress. And without them, resistance stretching cannot work. The stronger you are, and the better your cardiovascular capacity, the more you are able to challenge your body to work harder, longer, and faster when you stretch. Most resistance stretchers participate in some other form of regular exercise, from biking and running to swimming and weight training. Warning: Overtraining in any of these will defeat the effectiveness of the others.

Steam or dry heat your muscles

Some people prefer steam heat and others dry heat. Steam heat goes deep into your bones and takes stiffness and soreness out. Dry heat dries out your lungs and facilitates better oxygen absorption. Sweating in general should be viewed as a very good thing. The more you sweat, the healthier your skin is. Sweating also is usually a good indicator of a healthy immune system that can remove the waste products for any form of exercise. Remember, your skin is one of the three major elimination organs of your body. Steaming before or after stretching keeps muscles loose and limber. Steam baths, saunas, or even moderate hot-cold flush showers increase your core temperature and encourage circulation and lymph flow. These feed, clean, and massage your muscles and help to reduce soreness and hasten recovery.

Rest

Your body builds and repairs during rest, not during exercise. Getting the amount of sleep you need is imperative. A lot of people, including Lyndi and I, have found that going to bed by 9:30 P.M. and waking up at around 5:30 A.M. is the best regular schedule. This is not every night, but definitely most nights. Not everyone's lifestyle allows this, of course. Learn to do nothing. That means lying around and not doing anything. This is the only way you can recharge energetically. I'm not talking about listening to music or watching a movie. I'm talking about doing *absolutely nothing at all*—and for a good chunk of time, like twenty minutes or so. You can also do nothing for brief moments all day regardless of what is happening or whom you are with.

The comment I hear more than any other from new resistance stretchers is, "I can't believe what a good workout I'm get-

ting!" Even die-hard "alpha athletes" are unprepared for the level of exertion and energy resistance stretching demands. That's why it's so important to rest and rejuvenate your body afterward. Most resistance stretchers become masters of the quick nap. Doing nothing gives the body an opportunity to recharge like a battery, and it is essential to optimal performance.

You've built up a great stretching routine for yourself and you're loving how your body feels and your life is changing. And then—horrors!—you hit a roadblock, a tight spot you can't imagine how you're going to get yourself out of. Don't despair! We all come to points in our flexibility progress where we need guidance. Now I am going to share some troubleshooting techniques that will be sure to come in handy.

Troubleshooting Stretching and Helpful Hints

I would probably find you more perfect than you do. No, I'm not naïve. I've spent a lot of time helping people and I've seen everything under the sun. I'm always amazed by how much works correctly in everyone as opposed to how much works incorrectly in a body. But I also know that there are always a few things that just don't ever seem to work right in our bodies, and they are downright worrisome and frustrating. "If I could only be eighteen again," people say. I respond, "You are eighteen . . .

plus some other ages also. I can show you how to have a better body than you probably had at eighteen. You won't get everything you want from stretching, but you'll get plenty!"

You need to be really honest with yourself when you stretch. It's difficult to accept that you have problems in your body. But we all do. What you are looking for are the target areas of source tension. Once you find them, by stretching those areas, your whole body begins to unravel. After a while, you will feel free and trusting enough to ask for help.

When you first begin to stretch, you're not exactly a brand-spanking-new car. You have a little body work to do before you're working and feeling like new. The troubleshooting chart on page 255 can help you rebuild and upgrade your Maserati . . . and remember, it's never too late when it comes to stretching. Achieving the body you always imagined is much easier than you feared because of what we know about how to stretch. It's an analytical, targeted, logical, and willful process.

All of us have past physical injuries. Some you may remember vividly when you got them. Others may have happened so long ago that you aren't able to recall a particular incident except you've had this nagging and persistent pain that never seems to go away. These past injuries leave an imprint on your body. They are still making their presence felt—tugging and pushing on your muscles and surrounding tissues.

Other injuries may also be affecting your energy level or well-being. The good news is that stretching can dramatically improve, if not erase, a lot of the past damage.

You and I and everyone else have some "ketchup" to do. We need to restore our natural ranges of motion. In fact, we don't want simply to remove the restrictions. We want to advance forward, feeling better than we did before any damage occurred. It's important to face when things invariably go wrong in stretching. Denial only exacerbates things. Whether you are currently doing something wrong or have uncovered some problem you didn't know you had, you can assertively take the situation in hand and turn it into something really positive for yourself.

There are just a few simple ideas you need to grasp in order to help, correct, and reverse the damage of past injuries and advance beyond where you originally left off. These recommendations are not complicated—they are simple really.

You Need More Flexibility

When you are inflexible or have damage to even one muscle, the rest of your body compensates. Visualize your body as a webbed net of material. When an injury occurs, the net gets snagged toward the point of impact. The closer any part of your body is to the target area, the more warped or tightly wound that area becomes. Remove the dysfunction at the target source area, and the surrounding areas release as well (though they too will probably need some help if it has been a long time since the original injury occurred). One muscle in an area can create havoc with how your entire leg, arm, or torso moves. We'll call these target source muscles.

Example: You strained your right hamstring when you were running one day. Ever since then, your lower back hurts. You've tried abdominal strengthening exercises, which have given you some relief, but longer, more rigorous runs are impossible now. Remove the damaged tissue in your hamstring by using resistance stretching to stretch out the scar tissue, and your hip and thigh are no longer glued together. They are now moving freely with one another—connected but independent—the way they are supposed to be. Now when you move your leg, your lower back doesn't have to be yanked around by your hamstrings, and you're able to run pain free even when the run gets more challenging than before your injury. But you also can now run even better than before—faster, smoother, more effortlessly—and thus you love to run even more. Great!

You Need More Strength

When a muscle is inflexible, it is also limited in its ability to shorten. When you make certain movements that utilize that muscle, it is too weak to move your bones the way they need to move. So then other muscles try to compensate (this is called substitution). But substitution never works, because the wrong bones and joints are trying to do movements they are not really equipped to do. Troubled waters.

Example: You fell off a bike when you were very young. At the time, you probably cried a little and then got right back on. But now, years later, you subconsciously remember that spill whenever your knee bothers you or the weather changes or when you move just the "wrong" way. You have learned to be apprehensive about the way you move whenever your knee needs to bend in a certain way, and this is preventing you from maximal exertion or from putting everything into your favorite sport, soccer. In fact, your original accident actually resulted in a slight torque of your thigh on your lower leg, so now those two bones don't ever really align properly. The muscles on the inside of your thigh were damaged. For immediate relief, you go to a chiropractor whenever your knee starts to act up. But there appears to be no permanent escape from the problem. If you stretch the muscles on the inside of your thigh, voilà! Your thigh and lower leg are no longer misaligned. You lose your apprehension and those muscles can now contract, and because they are also more flexible, they now have the luxury of becoming stronger. You gain complete recovery, and you also move better than ever. Soccer goes up.

Your Body Is Too Toxic

You may have been too unhealthy or have been injured for too long. You body has become toxic, and this shows up as your body being too tough and rubbery, stiff, and too thin or fat. You no longer even have the option of doing many of the activities that you used to really like doing. First, you have to remove toxins, then you need to detoxify your body.

Stretching Snafus

You've been stretching for a while and are thrilled with the increases in your movement, elasticity, and range of motion. You're cruising along, no clouds on the horizon, and then, wham, something goes wrong. Suddenly your left thigh goes numb when you try certain stretches or your arm gets stuck, almost as if it has a hitch in it, or you have no leverage in your waist because your hips and lower back have unaccountably frozen on you.

What you could do before, now suddenly you can't. These stretching snafus are usually the result of some small, but easily modifiable, mistake that you've been making when you stretch. Or because stretching has made it possible for you now to do what was previously impossible, you have overdone it somehow.

The good news is that if you do things incorrectly, with a little guts and insight you can figure out how to do them correctly. If you have decided to try to improve the flexibility of some part of your body but something goes wrong, then all you have to do is figure out what you overlooked. You probably need to back up a little and let your body order you around (follow its lead instead of your lead), until you can feel what is causing what went wrong. You work on fixing the problem, and then you get to zoom ahead even more quickly. There will always be important things that you will overlook, but that's to be expected.

Mission Impossible

Things can be much more complicated than the previous examples present. Here are some other things to think about. The muscles of your upper body are supported by the structure of your lower body. Sometimes problems in your upper body originate from problems in your lower body, and vice versa.

Example: You have tennis elbow, experiencing inflammation of the tendons of the elbow caused supposedly by strain in repeatedly rotating your forearm. You have tried massage, strengthening exercises, and even stretching exercises (not resistance stretching yet) for the muscles that affect your elbow, but you've gotten no permanent relief.

Here's a thought: Your elbow muscle group is identical to the muscle group on your lower body that's on the outside of your hips. Try stretching out these lateral lower-body muscles, which seemingly have nothing to do with your elbow, and see if your elbow pain disappears into thin air. Though it is not always obvious how a problem in one area of your body can cause a problem in another part of the body, this is always happening. I'm hoping that you by reading this book you are learning how to make some of these connections.

Troubleshooting Principles

- Test your target muscle group for strength before trying to stretch. If these muscles are not strong enough, then strengthen first before stretching.
- Test your target muscle group's balancing muscle group's strength and flexibility. If these muscles need more strength or flexibility, develop them before stretching your target muscle group.
- Test the counterbalancing muscle group if your flexibility is not sustaining.
- You can be inflexible in the same muscle groups on both sides of your body (bilaterally inflexible), and you can be inflexible in the balancing muscle groups on the opposite sides of your body (asymmetrically inflexible). For example, your hamstrings on both sides of your body might need greater flexibility to become more bilaterally flexible, or your central hamstring on one leg and your central hip flexors on your other leg may need to be equalized in their flexibility. The

strategy is the same regardless—remove the inflexibility no matter where it is. You will have to spend more time removing chronic bilateral and asymmetrical inflexibilities by performing a large number of repetitions of the same stretches on whichever muscles are chronically inflexible until you have acquired the balanced flexibility that you desire everywhere.

- Consider whether you have enough food and water, as well as being rested enough before you begin.
- If your muscles don't readily stretch, you may need to detox yourself before you can ever possibly achieve the flexibility you desire.

Preventing Injuries

In order to be proactive about avoiding injuries, there are a few important rules to play by. You already know that you need to warm up sufficiently, to guard against going to extremes, and to be defensive when playing with others. But you need some additional advice to make a real difference in preventing injury. Here's the scoop on some great ways to stay out of trouble.

Stay balanced

By maximally resisting when you stretch, you know whether or not a muscle group can do what you need it to do. If it can resist maximally, you're all set. If not, you need to increase the flexibility of those muscles.

And remember, any muscle group that you need to stretch for an activity needs its balancing muscle group to be able to contract first. So when you need to stretch several groups of muscles for your particular activity, stretch the balancing groups first. For example, if you need flexible hamstrings for your chosen sport, then stretch your quads first. It's that simple.

Have the wind

Remember, when you do an energy stretch series, continuously sequencing from one stretch to another, you've got your aerobic exercise. This requires an aerobic capacity not usually experienced in most forms of traditional stretching. If you do all sixteen stretches and 6–10 reps of each stretch on both sides, then you just did 160 exercises in succession. That's not as aerobic as running or biking, but if you're stuck indoors, it's a great way to do aerobics. It's that simple.

Have the fuel

If you do not have great fuel and water stored in your body, then expect injury to chase after you when you exercise. Eating extremely fresh food and drinking unbelievably tasty spring water is the only way to go. Burn wet newspaper (fast food) or lubricate with toxins (soft drinks), and you make yourself a candidate for recycling, not competition. Remember, you are demanding

exceptional things of yourself, so an exceptional organic diet and whole-food supplements are a must. It's a great way to live.

Know about all four parts of yourself

You need to be aware of yourself physically, spiritually, emotionally, and psychologically. Even if you are stretching regularly, doing cardio regularly, weight training regularly, and eating good food regularly, all this can be erased in a single swoop if some other parts of your life are particularly dysfunctional. Any kind of self-defeating behavior can subtract from the benefits you're receiving.

The Straw That Broke the Camel's Back

Most injuries occur at some unusual moment. But where you became injured is more explainable than you might know. Most injuries occur to parts of your body that were already targeted areas of stress because of misalignments close by. For example, knees oftentimes become injured because of tightness of muscles around your hips that had prevented normal movements at your hips, and thus your knees found themselves doing jobs they were never intended or designed to do. So one day you do something that asks your hips to perform well, and instead, because they can't move well, your knees are asked to do the impossible—with the result that your knees get injured.

The logical preventive approach to avoid injures is to make sure your body can perform the movements that you want it to. Testing yourself in all sixteen different types of movements targets significant areas that need flexibility and/or strength. Go for it and develop your body so that you can have a really fun time doing what you like to do, and simultaneously reduce the possibilities of being injured.

Treating Injuries

Here are some great ways to fix yourself just in case you get in trouble. Fixing always takes three times the work as being preventive, but the solutions offered here are very doable—and hey, everyone makes mistakes, so be easy on yourself for whatever happened.

Warning: This chart assumes that you have had a knowledgeable health-care assessment and that you've decided to use noninvasive methods to rehabilitate yourself. If your injury is severe, be sure to consult a qualified health practitioner to assist you in the diagnosis, treatment, and recovery. The problems listed in this chart do not include severe muscle pulls, bone fractures or breaks, or severe physical damage to your body. The following is for the layperson to quicken recovery through stretching and strengthening. Seek other health professionals for solutions to more severe problems.

The following troubleshooting chart lists some of the most common problems, organized by your body parts. The first column lists your body parts. When you are experiencing a stress or injury somewhere in your body, look in the first column and find the body part that's affected. The second column lists common problems with that part of your body. Go down the list and locate your specific problem. The third column gives the recommended stretches or strengthening exercises that other stretchers with similar problems have found helpful.

Remember, in principle, the flexibility of any muscle depends on the flexibility of its balancing muscle group. The balancing group muscle is only as flexible as its ability to shorten sufficiently, which in turn is what allows your target muscle to get a really good stretch. Generally speaking, do not stretch any injured muscle. Instead, stretch all the muscles surrounding it; this changes the bone rotational relationships and takes stress off the injured muscle. If the muscle is strained, ice it until the swelling goes down, and then steam or dry heat it to speed recovery.

EXERCISE INJURY TROUBLESHOOTING CHART

BODY PART	PROBLEM	TARGETED STRETCH
Hip	Iliotibial strain	1, 2
	Iliopsoas strain	9, 10
	Gluteal strain	1, 2, 13, 14
	Piriformis issues	1, 2, 9, 10, 13, 14
Thigh	Adductor groin strain	1, 2, 5, 6, 13, 14
	Anterior thigh strain	5, 6, 9, 10
	Hamstring strain	1, 2, 9, 10, 13, 14
	Hamstring tendon problem	1, 2
Knee	Anterior cruciate ligament	1, 2, 9, 10, 13, 14
	Meniscus	15
	Medial collateral ligament	1, 2, 9, 10, 13, 14
	Lateral collateral ligament	1, 2, 9, 10, 13, 14
	Patella problem (jumper's knee)	9, 10, 13, 14
Lower Leg	Shin splints	5, 6, 9, 10
	Achilles tendon strain	9, 13
Ankle	Sprain (instability)	1, 2, 13, 14
Foot	Bunions	1, 2, 5, 6, 9, 10, 13, 14
	Plantar fasciitis	5, 6
Torso	Low back problems	1, 2, 5, 6, 9, 10, 13, 14
	Mid-back Problems	2, 7, 8
	Upper back problems	3, 4, 11, 12, 15, 16
Shoulder Girdle	Shoulder adductor strain	5, 6, 7
	Shoulder postural problems	3, 4, 5, 6, 7, 8
Shoulder Joint	Swimmer's shoulder	3, 4, 5, 6, 7, 8, 11, 12, 13, 14
	Limited external rotation dislocation	3, 4, 5, 6, 7, 8, 12, 13, 14
Upper Arm	Biceps strain	3, 11
	Triceps strain	4, 12
Elbow	Tennis elbow	6, 8, 11
	Golfer's elbow	2, 3, 6, 8, 11
	Surfer's elbow	3, 4, 5, 6, 7, 8, 9, 10, 11, 12
Forearm	Forearm strain	2, 3, 11, 12, 13
Wrist	Carpal tunnel	1, 2, 3, 4, 7, 8
Hand	Assisted stretches	See certified instructor
Neck	Stiff neck	4, 15, 16
Head	Head injuries	1, 4, 6, 8, 9, 12, 13, 16

Chapter 16

Stretching to Create Health and Prevent Illness

Heal yourself and others

ONE OF THE THINGS YOU BEGIN TO NOTICE with stretching is that there are subtle benefits that just kind of sneak up on you. When in repose—reading a book or watching a movie—you suddenly become aware of the rhythm of your breath, and it seems deeper and more natural to you. When you sit, you sit taller, straighter, and more assuredly. When you bend to pick something off the floor, suddenly the ground doesn't seem so far away. Driving in the car, you notice that the crink in your neck that you've had for the last fifteen years has disappeared. You turn your head, and there is fluidity and grace in your movement. When you've been engaged in a repetitive activity, such as sitting on your knees to weed the garden, instead of wincing when you stand back up, to your surprise your muscles and joints seem nonplussed. You can bounce back quicker, and ordinary activities become effortless and less conscious, freeing your mind for more important things. Life simply becomes more livable.

In the same way, stretching can be a great intercessor on our behalf. It protects and fortifies. If our bodies are like cars, then stretching is premium gasoline and a good tune-up! The following chart of common ailments and stretches can guide you to remove stresses in yourself that could evolve into more serious conditions over time.

The first column lists ailments by category. Go down the list and locate your specific problem. In the second column are stretches or strengthening exercises that other stretchers have found helpful in addressing similar problems, thereby upgrading their health. The categories include physical, physiological, tissue, illnesses, systems, psychological, and pregnancy.

If our recommendation in this health chart doesn't work, or if your problem is not listed, check out the Support option on our Web site for a much larger list of problems and solutions than provided here. www.MeridianStretching.com. Or you can e-mail us your question, and one of our great certified meridian flexibility trainers will e-mail you his or her recommendations, or you can use our weekly chat line to "Talk to Bob" in real time.

Note that the technical explanations for the recommendations in this chart are much more detailed than we can provide here. For a more exhaustive technical explanation, check out the *Meridian Flexibility Teachers Manual*, available for purchase on our Web site.

Remember that this book is not intended as a substitute for medical recommendations made by your health-care provider. Rather, it offers information to help you cooperate with your health-advancing experts, including alternative health-care providers, to gain optimum health. Please note that it is the expressed concern of the writer that all readers take responsibility for their health and for any and all advice they receive when engaging medical or health specialists.

PROACTIVE HEALTH CHART FOR RESISTANCE STRETCHERS

	STRETCHES
Physical Problems	
Achilles injury	9, 13
Ankle problems	1
Bunions	2, 6, 10
Carpal tunnel syndrome	11, 15
Elbow problems	2, 4, 7, 8
Foot problems	5, 6, 9, 10
Hand problems	3, 11
Hip problems	1, 2, 9, 10, 13, 14
Knee problems	1, 2, 6, 9, 13
Lower-back pain	1, 2, 5, 6, 9, 10, 13, 14
Muscle cramps	5
Muscle strain or sprain	5
Neck problems	1, 4, 9
Sciatica	1, 2, 9, 10, 13, 14
Scoliosis	1, 2, 9, 10, 13, 14
Shin splints	6
Shoulder problems	6, 7, 8, 11, 14
Swimmer's shoulder	7, 8
Tennis elbow	3, 4, 7, 8
Wrist problems	11, 15

STRETCHES

Physiological Problems

Appendix problems	4, 15
Bladder problems	13
Gallbladder problems	1
Heart problems	7
Internal immune problems	16
Kidney problems	14
Large intestine problems	4
Liver problems	2
Lung problems	3
Neurological (brain)	9
Pancreas problems	6
Pericardium problems	11
Small intestine problems	8
Sexual problems	10
Skin or external immune problems	12
Stomach problems	5

Tissues Concerns

Blood flow	7, 11
Bone	13
Cartilage ligaments	15
Cerebrospinal fluid	8
Fascia	6
Hormones	10
Joints	14
Muscles	5
Nerve tissue	13
Lymphatic flow	12
Lymph nodes	16
Organ linings	11
Oxygenation	3
Tendons	2
Venous flow	4

Illness and Disease

Acne	6
Appendicitis	15
Arthritis	6, 14

STRETCHES

Asthma	5
Bladder problems	13
Bronchitis (chronic)	3
Circulation	11
Colds	2, 3, 4, 5
Colon health	4
Constipation	4
Ear Infections	14
Eczema	6
Epstein-Barr	6
Fibromyalgia	6
Flatulence	1
Flu	11
Gallbladder conditions	1
Gum and tooth problems	6
Gynecological problems	10
Headaches	6
Heartburn	5, 6
Heart problems	7
Hemorrhoids	6, 9
High blood pressure	4
Kidney problems	14
Insomnia	7, 11, 12
Liver conditions	2
Menopause	9
Muscle pulls	5
Nervous system problems	9
Pancreas problems	6
Parasites	4, 6, 8, 15
Pericardium problems	11
PMS	6
Posture	all
Prostate problems	2, 13
Sexual problems	14
Sinus problems	10
Skin problems	12
Spleen problems	6, 16
Stomach problems	5
Thyroid	14
Toxic poisoning	4, 15

	STRETCHES
Vertigo	4, 6
Weight problems	14

System Concerns

Bones and skeleton	13
Cardiovascular system	3, 4
Central Nervous System	9
Connective tissue and fascia	6
Digestive	1, 2, 4, 5, 6
Endocrine system	14
External immune disorders	12
Integumentary system	12
Internal immune disorders	16
Joints	10
Lymphatic system	12
Metabolism	5
Muscle	5
Peripheral nervous system	9
Reproductive	10
Respiratory	3
Urinary system	13, 14

Psychological Concerns

Addictive	5
Anxious	2, 8, 10, 13
Avoidant	7
Borderline	14
Codependent	2
Depersonalized	15
Depressed	8
Distressed	15
Fearful	1, 5, 9, 14
Frightened	4, 6, 11, 15
Martyrish	6
Masochistic	11
Menticidal (brainwashing)	16
Narcissistic	13
Obsessive-compulsive	4
Overdependent	2

	STRETCHES
Panic attacks	11
Paranoid	9
Passive-aggressive	3
Sadistic	12
Schizoid	14
Stressed	12

Pregnancy Concerns

Childbearing	5, 6, 9, 10, 13, 14
Childbirth	6
Postpartum recovery	6, 13, 8

As you've seen in this chapter, stretching reaches into all corners of our well-being, placing the control of our internal and external health in our own capable hands. It's not easy to be the people we're intended to be when we're feeling stressed, or out of sorts, or just plain sick. With stretching in our medicine cabinet, so to speak, we have a safe and effective tonic that will help keep us fortified and fulfilled year after year. Now we're able to get more out of the things that bring us pleasure.

Stretching for Sexual Enhancement

I've worked with so many different people over the years who have shared their most intimate sexual stories with me that I have learned to value everyone's need to enjoy healthy and pleasurable sex lives. I know that some people don't have sex, but whether you are sexually active or not, I think you will find that this chapter has relevance . . . because it's really about complet-ing intimacy.

Sex is by definition a resistance stretch, because it involves very natural involuntary moments of tension and release, contrac-tion and relaxation. And just as with other resistance stretches, positioning, resistance, breathing, and psychological insight all play important roles.

You're probably thinking I'm going to talk about how being more flexible will allow you to get into many different posi-tions that you and your partner could not get into before you stretched. It's true that being flexible in your positioning can be an advantage. But increasing your flexibility positively affects your sex life not just by giving you better moves, so to speak. Stretching affects your sexual way of being, and this is about a lot more than finding the right positions. Let's look at the four aspects of greater intimacy, starting with the most seemingly obvious—the physical part.

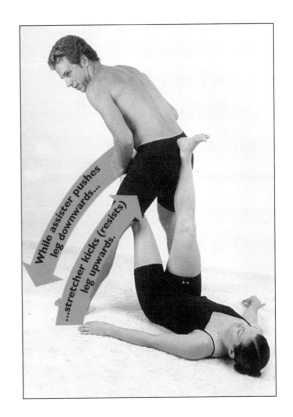

While assister pushes leg downwards...

...stretcher kicks (resists) leg upwards.

The physical part—lovemaking

Do you believe that when you were younger you had better sex than you do now? This may be true, but having great sex is not, and should never be, dependent on age. In fact, you should be getting better with age.

The physical part of sex revolves around your body and the act of making love. Developing your body obviously en-hances your physical appeal and your ability to be more natural and effortlessly physical when expressing yourself sexually.

For example, did you know that the muscles that contract involuntarily when you climax are located on the front and back inside of your pelvis? The muscles on the front are the iliopsoas and the muscles on the back are the six outward rotators. When you have sex, these muscles show you how to move your pelvis instead of using your lower back and front and back thigh mus-cles. This holds true for both men and women. You can increase the flexibility of these muscles only after stretching all the superficial muscles first.

The more flexible these muscles are, the more they can contract and the more you can move your hips. The result is greater variation in speed, direction, and the force you generate. No joke. People never believe me when I say that their orgasms will be better if they stretch these muscles. But they all go home and try it and come back to me saying, "Boy, were you right. Let's do some more of those!" These deep muscles are featured in Stretches 9 and 10.

That's just one of the many physical aspects of sex. Stretching also improves your skin, your physical appeal, and your ability to move. And all of the physical stretches improve your level of comfort during sex (and prevent cramps or back pain afterward).

It may be less obvious to you that *love* emerges from the physical part of yourself. Stretch 7 increases your ability to be romantic; stretch 3 accesses your feelings of vulnerability; stretch 12 increases your ability to role-play and reverse roles when being sexual; and stretch 15 shows you how to use sex to heal yourself and your partner.

This might seem enough in and of itself to ensure a great sex life. But you've only just begun! Now let's add the spiritual part and play with energy.

The spiritual part—bonding

Perhaps you wouldn't put "spirituality" and "sex" in the same sentence. But here again, I've listened to many real stories about how people's energies and lives and values have been affected through sex. Your sexual energy is your life force. The spiritual part of you determines your ability to communicate successfully, to bond in a monogamous relationship, to create a oneness with your partner, to be friends as well as lovers, to identify each other's individuality, to know when to control things and when to let go, to be open, to change, and to allow your imagination to go wild.

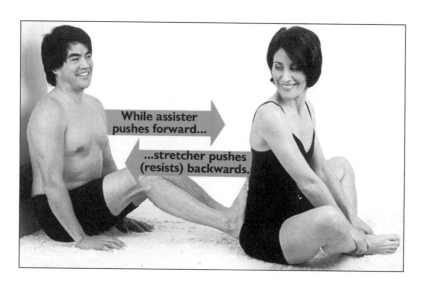

While assister pushes forward...

...stretcher pushes (resists) backwards.

When people first have sex, the newness of the experience brings with it an energy and unabashed spontaneity and curiosity that are unique and perhaps difficult to replicate in future relationships. But when we are sexually inexperienced, we don't typically show a lot of discernment in whom we choose to be intimate with. As you learn to value yourself and others more, you naturally become more selective with the partners you choose.

The impossible-to-put-into-words energetic sexual experiences that everyone has experienced are left for poetry in its highest forms. Entire religious traditions speak often of these states of ecstasy. Many tantric faiths expound on specific sexual techniques for elevating one's consciousness (e.g., Kama Sutra). Remember Sting's pronouncement that he had great sex by practicing yoga? It's wonderful for everyone to learn and explore this spiritual dimension.

Here are some stretches for developing the spiritual part of sex. To communicate successfully, to bond in a monogamous relationship, and to create a oneness, do stretch 6. To be friends as well as lovers, and to know when to control things and when not to, do stretch 4. To identify each other's individuality and to change, do stretch 15. And to become more open and have a wonderful sexual imagination, do stretch 11. All of the spiritual stretches increase your sexual energy.

These and other spiritual stretches allow you to develop the qualities of high regard, openness, and curiosity that are reflected in the ways you use your sexual energy.

The emotional part—
the act of caring

Emotional attunement has a lot to do with your ability to be intimate, accepting, and conscious of what you desire. The emo-

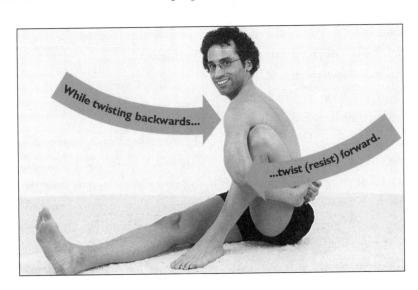

While twisting backwards...

...twist (resist) forward.

tional part of who you are controls your level of consciousness and is inseparable from the ways you allow yourself to breathe. A large part of being sexual has to do with allowing your unconscious to be involved in your sexual state of being and not controlling or even knowing what you are doing. Emotionality specifically affects your looks, your spontaneity and lack of inhibition, your performance and results, and your passion.

Stretching can improve your level of intimacy in a number of ways. Different stretches encourage you to confide to a close partner or friend your most intimate experiences. Having at least one person with whom you can share your sexual secrets is like inhaling pure oxygen. You feel fresh and accepted (and a little relieved) afterward. It doesn't matter what you did, and whether you thought it was good or bad; you need to hear yourself say it to someone close, someone you can trust. When you open up to that person, you might find that instead of being judged, you both end up laughing hysterically. Because invariably, your confidant has a few stories of his or her own. And pretty soon you're both on the floor laughing and begging each other to stop.

Communication is another big aspect of the emotional side of sexuality. You need to let your partner know when what he or she is doing is a "don't stopper" or if something needs to change. Some people communicate by physically moving their partner, who understands kinetic language better than verbal, while others need to talk to get things to happen in the right way. The inherent vulnerability in this level of openness requires that you transcend your self-consciousness and shyness, and learn how to express yourself openly and honestly. (It also helps to be diplomatic!)

Stretch 2 increases your ability to be less repressed; stretch 10 increases your capacity for compassion and acceptance; stretch 8 encourages you to be intensely passionate; stretch 13 keeps you on track so that you get the result you're looking for.

These four ways of being emotional with sex allow for greater responsiveness, the ability to climax, and the ability to lose the inhibitions and anxieties related to sexuality. Unresolved sexual issues usually have little to do with bedroom "gymnastics." They are often related to past traumas that are interfering with or blocking complete sexual growth and maturity. Learning to be emotional in these ways brings you a trustworthy, compassionate, and balanced partner.

The mental part—trusting

I hope your mind doesn't get up and leave the room when you're making love because it plays a huge role in your experience of intimacy. The mental dimension allows you to master your lovemaking skills; to be trusting, diplomatic, and loyal; to get something to happen; to persevere; to make a

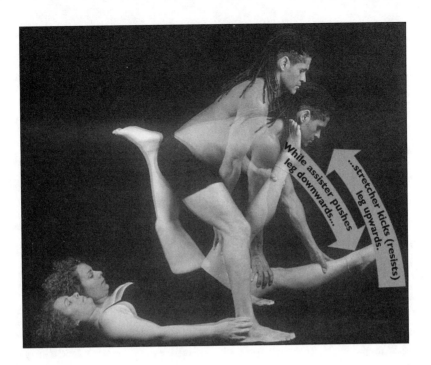

While assister pushes leg downwards...

...stretcher kicks (resists) leg upwards.

dance of sex; and to work through the relationship when it needs special attention.

For example, your ability to determine whom to trust and in what ways is essential for your safety in choosing partners. When you decide that you can trust your partner to honor your boundaries, this automatically leads to increased spontaneity. Any and all sexual traumas from your past will reenact themselves if they are not lifted out of you by some therapeutic means. Your loyalty to your partner and to yourself determines the freedom that is experienced in your relationship. Being sexual is not about being addicted to sex. Being sexual involves embracing just the right amount of sex in your life and understanding that it is a lot of work, in the most positive sense of that word. The depth and understanding of your

partner are critical in determining the outcome of your moments of intimacy.

To increase your feelings of trust and to master your lovemaking skills, do stretch 9. To be more loyal and devoted, do stretch 1. To get things started, to make a dance of sex, to enjoy working at it, to increase your self-expression, and to get what you wish for, do stretch 5. To increase your sensory awareness, simply to stay in the moment of being sexual (instead of being anxious for the result), and to experience sexually cathartic experiences, do stretch 14.

Your psychological health allows you and your partner to enjoy all aspects of each other's personalities when being sexual. The growth of your mental functions depends on how you use your sexual energy. Your brain literally needs sexual energy as its fuel, so to speak. So developing free-flowing sexual feelings brings a much-needed intelligence into your lovemaking. The mental part gives you access into the totality of being sexual.

Change and De-toxing

Reaching critical mass

The best investment in your flexibility is great nutrition. When you have been too inactive or injured, or have been eating not particularly wonderful food (understatement of the century) over a long period of time, then you need to remove the toxins and detox. Your body is filled with toxins even if you ingested those icky things twenty-plus years ago. When you are too full of toxins, your body reacts like it was bitten by a poisonous snake—every muscle stays contracted. It's really that bad. Do not procrastinate—begin to detox now. Remember, denial comes with too much fat; they are stuck together.

When you began stretching, you, like everyone, else found that resistance stretching gave you immediate, cumulative, and permanent changes in your flexibility. Then suddenly the gains you were making in flexibility stopped. What happened? Your inability to make continuing flexibility gains is probably not a result of stretching incorrectly. It is not your fault that you suddenly find your flexibility going backward instead of forward. You have reached a point where you are or have become internally too toxic, and just like someone who has been poisoned, your body begins to cramp and tighten instead of continuing to loosen.

Your body has not been removing the waste products that are a natural by-product of stretching and exercise. So you fill with these waste products and all the tissues of your body slowly become poisoned. The tissue in your arms and legs and torso begins to feel hard and rubbery, stiff and dry, brittle, with a dense outer layer of fat. No matter how much stretching you do, or aerobic exercise, steaming, or massage, these negative qualities about your body stay pretty much the same—or become worse.

How to fast correctly

Not eating is not what fasting is about. Not eating is starving yourself and is quite dangerous. Fasting correctly involves removing any parts of regular foods that cause your body to have an appetite. Therefore, daily consumption of strained vegetable and fruit broths keeps your body nourished, to keeps you from feeling weak, prevents you from craving solid food, and makes you feel incredible.

I am no authority on fasting. Instead, I refer you to these organizations which can guide you through your fast and are in my opinion, an indispensable partners when fasting. Here's how to contact them:

Fasting Center International
27C East Victoria
Santa Barbara, CA 93101
www.fasting.com

www.mercola.com

The benefits of fasting

All the parts of your body that you probably hate the most are what fasting removes first—excess fat, old scar tissue, and tough connective tissue. And while all this excess baggage is melting away, you are not losing much muscle, not feeling particularly weak, and instead are becoming incredibly clear-minded, as flexible as a baby, with skin and hair to die for.

Why does your body do this? It's quite simple. When you fast, your body immediately prioritizes what to save for survival and what is expendable. So for fuel, while fasting, your body burns up the expendables: excess fat, old scar tissue, and tough connective tissue.

Say good-bye to your spare tire of fat
Who would ever guess that the spare tire around your waist is what your body likes to eat first when you fast? Or those saddle bags hanging on the sides of your upper thighs.

Nonsurgical removal of scar tissue and tough connective tissue
Who could ask for more? As your body eats up old scar tissue and pounds of thick tough connective tissue that were encircling your muscles like bullies, not allowing your muscles to move, you are turning into Gumby.

Increased circulation everywhere
Who wouldn't like his or her hands and feet to be nice and toasty warm all year? That's right, fasting increases circulation every-where, even within your insides around your organs.

Your skin daily gets more and more incredible
Say good-bye to pimples and bumpy skin and hello to silky, translucent, and tight skin. Your immune system is composed of miles of moving lymph that removes junk from your skin. Steam or dry saunas will help to empty your skin of old bad stuff.

Your metabolism corrects itself
If your metabolism was too slow before your fasted, after your fast it speeds' up. And if your metabolism was too fast before you fasted, then it slows down. Could you ask for more? I don't think so.

Chapter 17

The Organic Lifestyle

Ending the stigma of organic

SEVERAL MONTHS AFTER BEGINNING TO STRETCH, a friend noticed that we were both buying only organic food. We had quietly and unconsciously slipped into choosing only "certified organic," not because we knew anything about it or thought it was better for us but because we simply felt more nourished when we ate certified organic food. We found that we ate smaller quantities of food yet had greater satisfaction. It seemed to be a logical, natural extension of the stretching experience.

Only years later did I begin seeking out organic everything: cotton and wool clothing, housewares, furniture, and other products. Still later did I discover nontoxic paints and compost, and nonpaper copy paper. Ten years later, I was attending organic conferences, making friends with owners of organic companies, tending my own organic garden, and developing global views about sustainable everything. I had stretched myself back into my body and out into the world, and now I found that organic resonated with everything I had learned about stretching. I couldn't have been more delighted than to meet the parents of Olympic athlete Eli Fairfield, who raised him on an organic farm. All of the Olympic athletes I work with now are eating organic and eagerly embracing a world of sustainable resources, a reflection of their own healthy, sustainable bodies. If your stretching is organic, then why wouldn't your food and everything else become organic also? This is a natural progression.

Why Organic, Sustainable, Fair Trade, Local, and Recycle

The basic principles behind certified organic outline that you buy much of your food locally (and in season), and that whoever helps you to live must be paid fairly for spending his or her life feeding, clothing, or otherwise contributing to your life. Staying connected to all the people in your life who make your life possible not only lifts your integrity but also helps you to live the philosophy that everything is connected. Allow your awareness to embrace this global perspective. And remember to recycle everything.

This is a huge topic, and there's way too much to talk about to do it justice in this chapter, so I'll refer you to sources that can

Dare to make life for everyone on our planet always better than you can imagine.

help to educate you about organic living. Please check out:

Organic Trade Association: www.ota.com
International Federation of Organic Agriculture Movements: www.ifoam.org
Ecology Action: www.growbiointensive.org

Many of the organic products that I recommend are available at Jimbo's, Whole Foods, Wild Oats, and Alfalfa Grocery stores as well as other organic specialty stores. If you don't have these stores near you, nearly all retail grocery chains have some organic selections. Once you've filled up your cart with all these goodies, you'll probably be grateful for a few suggestions on what kinds of meals to prepare. This chapter shows you how to eat and where to buy everything organic. I've also included sample breakfasts, lunches, dinners, and snacks to get you started and to introduce you to the delicious options that will assuredly point you down the organic food path.

Warning: Once you begin eating certified organic food, you'll want everything else in your life to be organic: your socks, your sheets and blankets, your cleaning products, your paint, your partner . . .

Nutrient-Rich Foods and Flexible Meals

All the people I've taught to stretch begin to buy and prefer fresh organic foods (if they

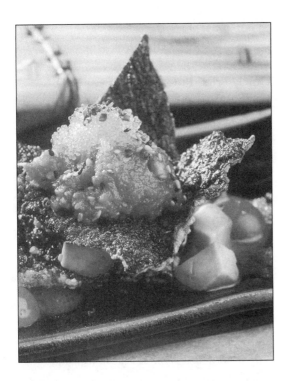

stuffed down their throat. I like restaurants that let you make substitutions so you can have the meal your body really craves at that moment and aren't forced to follow some arbitrary "food policy." I give you several options for each meal, because, after all, making your own choices is what flexible eating is all about! Mix the entrees, side dishes, salads, and desserts to suit your needs. And of course the meals are quick and simple to make.

If you can also eat food that naturally grows where you are in each season, you'll find that your body really likes these foods and appreciates that you've decided to feed yourself for each season.

Nutrient-rich food supplements like Living Fuel's Very Berry Drink are certified organic and wild harvested (this company also has the best omega 3s you'd ever desire). Take only food-based vitamins. One more thing: Eat fresh food. The freshest food is picked just before you eat it. The fresher the food, the more nutritious it is. For example, salad greens that are literally just picked from a garden and eaten within minutes digest almost instantly like they were liquids. I recommend that you spend the extra time and effort to eat fresh—nothing is better. Yes, no matter where you live, create an organic garden and make your own compost.

I'm getting hungry just thinking about it. So let's eat . . .

weren't already doing so). Then they always want to know what they should eat! It wouldn't be fair if I didn't share with you some of my favorite all-organic meals and recipes.

What follows are samples of everything organic meals (including snacks). I list some terrific cookbooks after this sampler, some written by my friends who are organic chefs. These books are fun and creative, and they show you how easy and satisfying it is to eat well and healthy. If you are "kitchen challenged," their books also provide everything you need to know, step by step.

I believe that people who are described as fussy eaters simply are not given enough choice in what they eat. It's not that they're fastidious so much as that everyone else is being inflexible. Food is literally being

Organic Breakfasts

Before or after your morning stretch.

- Preparation for most meal options is within 15 minutes.
- Presoak precooked grains overnight and prepare in advance of the meal.
- Portion size is to your discretion.
- Basic cooking directions are included.

Option 1

Two Organic Free-Range Eggs
Cook any way you like.

Organic Buttermilk Pancakes with Organic Butter, Blueberries, and Maple Syrup
I like Arrowhead Mills Buttermilk Pancake Mix.

Mixed Sautéed Vegetable Stems
Chop beet, kale, collard, or chard stems (or a combo) into small pieces, then sauté in organic olive oil with tamari.

Spring Water or Organic Tea

Option 2

Small Piece of Organic Beef with Snow Peas
Pan-sear beef strips in a little butter and mango or orange juice. Add snow peas and a touch of spring water and sea salt.

Sautéed Arugula in Organic Olive Oil with Nonpasteurized Tamari

Stir-fry arugula, oil, and tamari for 2–3 minutes.

Quick-Fried Potato Sticks with Sea Salt
Slice baked potatoes into sticks. Pan-fry with oil and salt.

Spring Water or Organic Tea

Option 3

Small Piece of Wild Coho Salmon
Broil salmon with basil; add lemon.

Fried Quinoa with Onion, Carrot, and Celery Pieces
Soak quinoa overnight so that it begins to sprout. Pan-fry with onion, carrot, and celery pieces in organic olive oil.

Peas with Organic Butter
Boil peas for a short while with butter.

Sliver of Fruit Tart
Place selected fruits in an organic whole wheat pastry crust; add maple syrup. Bake for 35 minutes.

Spring Water or Organic Tea

Option 4

Quinoa Rice and Scrambled Eggs with Sautéed Onion, Fresh Corn, and Cherry Tomatoes
Mix precooked quinoa, scrambled eggs, and sautéed vegetables, then add tomatoes.

Sautéed Beet Tops
Chop beet stems. Pan-fry with olive oil and tamari.

Organic Jewel Dates
Spring Water or Organic Tea

Option 5

Organic Granola or Warm Quinoa with Organic Monnuka Raisins, Organic Coconut, and Organic Walnuts
Goatein Banana Smoothie or Living-Fuel "SuperFood" Drink
Blend a banana and other fruits with 2 tablespoons of Goatein.

Spring Water or Organic Tea

Organic Lunches

Your midday energy boost fortifies your for the rest of the workday without making you feel sluggish and dull.

- Lunch can be light or dinnery.
- Do what works for you.
- If you're eating with other people (always a good idea), let everyone eat different food.

Option 1

Fresh Picked Mesclun Mix and Cherry Tomato Salad, with Olive Oil and Brown Rice Vinegar
Mix everything together. Add your own preferred fresh or dried herbs—oregano, basil, thyme.

Baked Chicken Thigh with Thyme, Lemon, and Honey
Bake chicken thigh with selected herbs.

Organic Brown Rice with Zucchini Strips
Sauté zucchini strips and garnish over rice.

Spring Water

Option 2

Fresh-Picked Basil, Heirloom Tomatoes, and Organic Mozzarella and Organic Olive Oil
Layer tomatoes, cheese, and basil, drizzle on oil.

Small Piece of Wild Coho Salmon on Fresh-Picked Romaine Leaves
Broil salmon. Sprinkle on fresh basil. Place on top of romaine lettuce leaves.

Steamed Veggies
Steam carrots, beets, and other root vegetables.

Maple Syrup–Sweetened Cornbread with Fresh Corn
I like Arrowhead Corn Bread Mix: substitute organic barley malt, organic maple syrup, or organic date sugar for sweetener.

Spring Water

Option 3

Organic Lamb with Organic Celeriac, Organic Butter, and Organic Elephant Garlic
Pan-sear lamb with butter, small celeriac pieces, and garlic.

Quinoa and Brown Rice

Sautéed Beet Stems and Collard Greens
Sauté beet, collard, etc., stems in organic olive oil with a dash of sea salt.

Sliver of Date-Sweetened Carrot Cake
I enjoy the carrot cake recipe in Moosewood Cookbook.

Spring Water

Option 4

Fresh Vegetable Juice
Use Brand Juicer with vegetable(s) of your choice.

Sprouted Flat Bread with Olive Oil and Organic Cheese
Heat Ezekiel Sprouted Flat Bread in oven or toaster. Drizzle with olive oil and top with a slice of organic cheese.

Oatmeal Cookie
I like the recipe in Lake House Cookbook: *Substitute organic date sugar for sweetener.*

Spring Water

Option 5

Stir-Fried Vegetables with Broiled Tofu, Ginger, and Tamari
Broil tofu with ginger, basil, and tamari. Mix with stir-fried veggies.

Micro Green Salad
Microsprouts can be found in your organic grocery. Select greens that tickle your

fancy. Toss with olive oil and a very subtle dressing.

Spring Water

Snacks or Meal Supplements

Satisfy the munchies with foods that build you up rather than tear you down. Try the Organic Food Bars (they have no refined sugar). This is the best time of day to eat vine-ripened fruit. You might also need another Goatein Smoothie by GardenofLife .com, a Super Berry Drink from Living Fuel.com, or Cocochia, which is organic coconuts and chia seeds.

Organic Dinners

Reward your body after your workout and give it something good to dream on . . .

- Dinner is best before 7 P.M. so you have time to digest before sleeping.
- Go light or full based on your needs.
- Don't eat alone too often; you digest better with close friends.

Option 1

Broiled Organic Beef with Mango
Marinate tenderloin in mango juice, then broil.

Mesclun Salad
Create the mixed green salad of choice. Dress organically.

Artichoke Heart with Organic Butter

Steam artichokes. Serve with butter.

Organic Yam Mashed Potatoes

Bake yams. Mash with butter.

Spring Water

Option 2

Lamb with Thyme, Butter, and Garlic

Bake lamb with herbs.

Organic Purple Potatoes with Peas and Organic Butter

Bake the potatoes with the lamb. Cover with buttered steamed peas.

Caesar Salad

Mix romaine or red leaf lettuce with fresh dressing—see Cooking with Nora.

Spring Water

Option 3

Chicken Vegetable Soup

Make stock—boil whole chicken with breasts, legs, and wings removed. Strain and remove excess fat. Sauté vegetables of choice; add to stock.

Organic Cornbread

I like Arrowhead Mills Corn Bread Mix. Substitute sweeteners.

Small Baby Green Salad
Spring Water

Option 4

Vegetable Stir-Fry on Fresh Lettuce

Pan-fry vegetables with tofu or tempeh. Serve on lettuce.

Avocado with Olive Oil and Brown Rice Vinegar

Slice avocado in shell. Add oil and vinegar.

Fresh Peas and Butter

Boil fresh peas with butter.

Spring Water

Option 5

Broiled Fresh Local Fish

Broil local fresh fish of choice with herbs.

Steamed Carrot Sticks

Quinoa and Brown Rice Vegetable Stir-Fry

Stir-fry vegetables. Add to prepared quinoa and rice.

Arugula Sautéed in Olive Oil and Tamari
Spring Water

Recommended Dietary Supplements

Very Berry Drink, Cocochia, Vitamins D and A, Omega 3's by LivingFuel.com

Primal Defense by GardenofLifeUSA.com

B Complex by NewChapter.com

Digestive Enzymes by Metagenitics.com

Calcium-Potassium by Metagenitics.com

Vitamin C Chewables by RainbowLight.com

Cooking Creatively

Books by the Best Organic Chefs

Here are some of my favorite cookbooks, some by my best friends.

Cooking with Nora by Nora Pouillon (Random House, 1996)

Your Organic Kitchen: The Essential Guide to Selecting and Cooking Organic Foods by Jesse Ziff Cool (Rodale, 2000)

Nourishing Traditions: The Cookbook That Challenges Politically Correct Nutrition and the Diet Dictocrats by Sally Fallon (New Trends Publishing, 1999)

The New Moosewood Cookbook by Mollie Katzen (Ten Speed Press, 2000)

The Whole Foods Market Cookbook: A Guide to Natural Foods with 350 Recipes by Steve Petusevsky (Clarkson Potter, 2002)

Healing with Whole Foods: Asian Traditions and Modern Nutrition by Paul Pitchford (North Atlantic Books, 2002)

The Lake House Cookbook by Trudie Styler and Joseph Sponzo (Clarkson Potter, 1999)

Where to Find the Ingredients for These Meals

The Resources section lists some companies that grow or produce the foods that are featured in these sample meals. Please give these companies your business. When you do, you help to set nutritional standards not just for yourself, but for the entire globe.

Seasonal Eating

Spring

This is the beginning of the new year. You have just finished detoxing and fasting, and now it is time to begin a new year's worth of eating great food. Renew yourself as spring presents itself in all its excitement. Spring is the time of year to fast. Nutrient-rich vegetable broths and juices comprise the best fasting.

In folk cultures around the world, green is the color that signifies spring. Dark, leafy greens are not only extremely low in calories, but they are also packed full of hundreds of phytonutrients, vitamins A and C, and minerals including potassium, magnesium, iron, and calcium. Other green foods abundant in the spring are scallions, artichokes, asparagus, fava beans, peas, pea shoots, and green garlic. These foods also are high in phytonutrients, vitamins, and minerals.

Nongreen spring fruits and vegetables include certain citrus fruits (most notably blood oranges and Meyer lemons), morels, papayas, and rhubarb. Strawberries are in season, but it is very important that you eat only organic strawberries. In a study by the Environmental Working Group, 90 percent of nonorganic strawberries tested were found to have residues from one or more of thirty-six different pesticides!

Seafoods such as soft-shell crabs, clams, grouper, catfish, halibut, shad and its roe, and salmon are in season in the spring and should be in abundance at your local seafood counter. Lamb and veal are also available, but make sure you purchase your meats from a trusted farmer who raises them humanely and without any hormones or antibiotics.

Summer

Summer is a season of outdoor activity and sunshine. Crops and plants naturally mature during this period, following the birth and growth characterized by the spring. So which foods do we eat to stay in balance with this active, dynamic season? Just look at the bounty of fresh fruits and vegetables available in summer to know how to keep cool during the long lazy days at the beach or on the lake.

Eggplant, corn, zucchini, all kinds of tomatoes and peppers, cherries, raspberries, peaches, plums, grapes, and watermelons begin to ripen in the summer, and you will likely find that your local farmer has these items available in abundance. Cold soups, salads, salsas, and fruits are good choices in the summer. Cucumbers are especially crisp, hydrating, and cooling—the epitome of the qualities we naturally gravitate toward this time of the year.

Both tomatoes (cooked) and water-melon are rich sources of lycopene, a potent antioxidant that has been shown to prevent prostate cancer. Other summer fruits are also nutritional powerhouses. Apricots, plums, and nectarines are full of vitamins A and C, potassium, and various phytonutrients. Cherries are high in an enzyme that neutralizes uric acid, which causes gout; they have been a favorite folk remedy for this condition for generations. Berries are packed with fiber, vitamins, minerals, and potent antioxidants.

You will probably be attracted to raw, lightly steamed, or quickly grilled vegetables during this time of year, when our bodies need lighter foods to counteract the hot and humid weather. We naturally slow down in the summer, so our bodies require light meals that are easy to digest and metabolize. Raw foods in particular are packed with beneficial digestive enzymes, which are mostly destroyed in the process of cooking.

Optimal summer menus include fresh local fruits and vegetables along with beans, nuts, seeds, and seasonal proteins—such as soft-shell crabs, halibut, lobster, and other available lean proteins—and, of course, lots of high-quality filtered water! Grilling is also a favorite mode of summer cooking. For healthy grilling, choose lean meats. High-temperature grilling produces carcinogenic compounds in the meat, so a better option is to grill over a low fire and use a meat thermometer to determine when the meat is fully cooked. Marinades with citrus, garlic, and turmeric are also believed to in-

hibit the cancer-causing substances produced when grilling meat. Whether you
have a barbecue or a picnic, or just take
your lunch to the park, dining outside is one
of the best ways to approach seasonal eating
this time of year.

Fall

Fall is a time of abundance, thankfulness,
and activity. Many cultures have their own
celebrations in the fall in which the community comes together to harvest food for
the winter. Fall provides us with a wide variety of items, since many summer and winter
crops are generally available at this time as
well.

When I think of fall produce, I think
of apples, pears, cranberries, mushrooms,
cauliflower, leeks, corn, lima beans, and the
glorious sweet vegetables—butternut, ka-
bocha, and acorn squashes, which are related to the most popular autumn treat,
pumpkins. Succotash beautifully illustrates
the earthy tones of fall food colors—yellow
corn and orange carrots with a smattering
of light green for the lima beans. These colors signify qualities of ripeness, maturity,
and decline. The orange flesh of autumn
foods—including carrots, squashes, and
sweet potatoes—indicates that they are very
high in vitamin A and potassium. Mushrooms are a surprisingly good protein
source, so vegetarians should certainly be
incorporating this food into their diet, especially in the fall. Mushrooms also contain
iron, thiamine, riboflavin, and niacin.
There is evidence to support the folk wisdom that certain mushrooms protect
against cancer.

A great way to take advantage of autumn vegetables is by preparing them in
soups. Simply chop whatever vegetables
you find at your local farmers' market, sauté
them in a small amount of olive oil, and
simmer until tender with sea salt to taste.
Add fresh seasonal herbs such as tarragon,
sage, rosemary, thyme, parsley, or cilantro
just before serving for an extra-special treat.

Maple syrup is a great seasonal sweetener to complement your grains and other
foods when you desire a sweet touch. The
sap of the maple tree turns sweet during the
fall, when it is harvested and boiled down
into syrup—sixty gallons of sap produce a
gallon and a half of syrup. Ounce for ounce,
maple syrup has more calcium than milk!
But, as with any sweetener, use it sparingly.
You will find it a delightful addition to the
autumn diet, especially as a replacement for
refined white sugar in recipes.

Game birds including pheasant, turkey,
and quail are appropriate sources of protein
during the fall season. If you hunt, or know
a hunter, this is a good way to indulge in
game birds. Alternatively, find a farmer who
raises them in a sustainable manner. Both
are good ways to align your protein consumption with what's available seasonally in
your area.

Winter

There's no easier way to start shopping than choosing foods that are in season and local. Just as bears hibernate and plants die down for the winter, humans have their own unique way of winding down during the colder, darker months. Seasonal winter foods are hearty, building foods, to ensure that we survive and remain healthy during this time of natural repose. Our bodies also require optimal nutrition to keep our defenses strong during the inevitable cold and flu season.

Winter produce consists of hardy vegetables such as brussels sprouts, cabbage, endive, escarole, leeks, kale, collard greens, parsnips, turnips, yams, rutabagas, and potatoes. These high-fiber foods keep our digestion running smoothly while our increased fat and protein needs are met on our winter diet. Heavier meats, including beef and pork, help sustain us through these months.

Dried fruits are also great winter foods, packed with fiber, B vitamins, and iron. They are highly concentrated sources of vitamins and minerals, so a little dried fruit goes a long way. Most citrus fruits are also in season, providing us with an extra dose of much-needed vitamin C.

Whole grains including spelt, kamut, oats, and barley are also winter staples. They are packed with B vitamins, minerals, and fiber. Hot cereal made with a whole grain is a versatile breakfast treat any time of the year but is especially nourishing in the winter. Add toasted nuts or seeds, dried fruit, and a natural sweetener such as maple syrup or honey, and you have a hearty, nutritious breakfast. You can also serve the grains as a side dish, in soups and stews, or even in desserts such as puddings and cobblers.

Stews, casseroles, and slow-braised foods are appropriate main dishes for the winter, as they provide the hearty stick-to-your-ribs feeling that is comforting as we retreat from the outside world (physically as well as mentally). Think of healthy foods that provide comfort and warmth when planning your winter menus.

Winter is a time for reflection and rest, and the winter diet perfectly complements that need to slow down, turn inward, reflect, and dream so that we are ready to extend outward—like plant shoots from the soil—when spring arrives!

Seasonal eating, facilitated by the consumption of locally grown organic produce, restores our natural sense of rhythm and balance. Don't be surprised if a transition to seasonal, whole foods restores your own equilibrium—bringing you better sleep, steadier moods, and vibrant energy!

You will also be participating in building a viable alternative to the current industrial food system, one in which food quality and the environment are valued, rural regions thrive, and ties between producers and consumers are strong. It would be nothing short of a food revolution!

Afterword

Whether we know it or not, we all try to re-create ourselves—to manifest the full value of ourselves. Every famous star knows they must subtly re-create themselves by becoming not just physically more appealing, but by becoming more developed psychologically, more mature emotionally, and more spiritually "zenithed." All these re-creations bring about a new "look" or persona that, in turn, catalyzes an avalanche of change in their lives, in their future endeavors, and in their breadth of appeal.

Evolving and investing in yourself increases your appeal and viability. Efforts to do just this dramatically increase your magnetism. When you re-create yourself from the inside out, your best qualities come forth, presenting themselves as a personality that just glows.

Resistance stretching absolutely re-creates everyone as they consciously select some aspect of themselves that they want to develop. Yes, their natural good looks most definitely come forth because the subtle internal changes in them have been extraordinary. Stretching is really more of a subtractive technology—it's more about taking stuff away, like weeding a garden so that the plants can thrive. And it's also about building yourself to include all the possible parts of yourself—bringing yourself into full splendor.

When you stretch, re-creating yourself will become a daily occurrence. Things that you have always wanted for yourself will come forth and grow and develop. Some things will change unexpectedly, while other things you'll tackle and the changes will flow. Some aspects of yourself take considerable effort to change, while other aspects will change quite easily. You decide what part of you that you want to re-create.

There are sixteen types of things to change. You simply practice the type of stretch that corresponds to those traits. In time, you will re-create yourself in surprising ways.

When You First Began . . .

When you first start stretching you are very grateful that your usual aches and pains begin to be subtracted from your normal awareness of your body. You also learn how by simply reversing the movements you do when you stretch, you can also strengthen any muscle. As you continue to stretch, you begin to understand how you are unwinding chronic tenseness out of yourself. You usually start feeling like you're getting some "things" that you have always wanted—a better shape, or better looking, or healthier in a particular way—or some specific psychological change has occurred, such as you become more sober, better at relating, more social, or have better judgment.

Soon you move from sporadic stretching into a regular daily stretching practice, and occasionally you even get a little intense about the way you stretch. You can now do end-position yoga postures that you previously thought were impossible. Many people like yourself had given up on yoga because they could never get into the more advanced positions. Now you get there daily. You've found a community of individuals who share and understand the value in the changes you all are making. Everyone is compassionate about your efforts, problems, and successes. A unique extended family has been ushered into your life.

You have quickly learned from innumerable and repeated experiences that you can remove your chronic aches, pains, and rusty joints forever. You wouldn't expect anything less from your stretching. What started out as a general increase in awareness of your body turns into awareness targeting specific problems. For example, when I first started to stretch, I discovered how to stretch the muscles on the back of my thighs. But several years later, I could differentiate the three different hamstrings on the back of my thigh, and how to stretch each of them specifically. Heaven *is* on earth.

When It Got Intense and Everything Started to Change . . .

Now you can stretch really intensely for a good hour and a half or more and you yearn for the improvements—your stretching has become turbocharged, making you feel light and strong. You no longer merely settle for an elevated mood and a better face and body. You're seeking dramatic changes in many aspects of yourself and in your life. This new intensity, though thrilling, also turns you a little inside out and upside down—literally! Sometimes it is like you have been operated on, only you're the surgeon. You're feeling new but somewhat disoriented. The people who assist you have become indispensable. You can't wait to get together with them.

⁓

My life is reflected in my body.
The world is reflected in my body.
Anyone can change the world.

⁓

You positively love the recent extraordinary changes in yourself. Your posture and movements have become more graceful, powerful, and exact. You express yourself and communicate with others a million times more effectively. Your mood is high but stable, but it's also loaded with fluctuations. Your feelings of self-worth and self-esteem couldn't be better. All the psychological frontiers are open. The gateway to the spiritual world has been crossed. Energy becomes almost palpable.

But nothing, and I mean nothing, in your life is staying much the same. And as long as you keep stretching intensely and regularly, the rate of all these changes keeps accelerating. However, there is also an ever-increasing peacefulness, calmness, stillness, and quietness about you. Everyone notices it, because they say you affect them that way. You probably would have never guessed that anyone would ever describe you as being this way. You are literally *being* in ways that would have been *a real stretch for you to be* in the past.

And what about other people? Well, people don't look the same to you anymore. You don't feel or think about other people in the same way either. The truth is you've learned how to value the best in others, and you intentionally bring out what you admire most about them, and in doing so you get to learn how to *be* in all the ways you've always wanted to be.

These new feelings and thoughts about people include your partner, your family, your friends, the people you work and play with, and everyone else you see even casually on the street, at restaurants, at the movies—everywhere. As a matter of fact, you have found yourself connecting and staying connected with everyone. You now think in global terms about everything.

⁓

Resistance stretching pulls you
together not apart
It's pulling your world together,
And you feel like pulling the world together.
Stretching requires your genius
And thus brings it out of hiding-forever.

⁓

You have learned how to identify in yourself exactly what others are feeling, and you can find your way out of their stuff and so guide them out of their mess. You also have learned that you need to know how to defend yourself from their snafus while doing this. You feel things that most people commonly overlook. Others' thoughts, feelings, intentions, and their pasts and futures become things you feel and imagine. You literally envision events and people that have or will occur to others and yourself. Your energetic perceptions bring with them the possibility for you to perform many kinds of unspoken actions—miracles.

From stretching you've learned that you need to feel and be the opposite of those bad feelings before you can go *underneath* them and raise them from within yourself, up and out forever—epiphanies. You've learned that being attached is as good as being detached; being physical is as good as being spiritual; that instincts are as good as knowledge; that analysis as good as logic; and that being subjective is as good as being objective. You have learned that at any one moment the past, future, and present are all reflected in the state of your body. You've learned that fear, anger, suffering, and anxiety are the negative sides of instincts that you've learned to process through (and not repress)—that it's essential to do this to change. As the awareness of these instincts guides you into the right actions to take, you quickly find yourself fearless, loving, alive, and excited. And you've learned to do this awareness-processing "trip" whether you or someone outside you is experiencing them. You have learned to turn (not repress) negative feelings and emotions into their opposites—like turning food waste into compost into rich soil that produces the best food—turning them into the best character traits known to humanity.

And your mind works like it's a room
full of people in a think tank,
Except they are all in one head—yours.

Ultimately, what you experience about yourself and others while you practice stretching begins to happen all day. The different ways you have learned to *be* while stretching, allow you to be very *flexible* in the way you are with yourself and others at any moment. Your physical side is about health, the thinking side of you is about knowing, your spiritual side is about living, and your emotional side is about being. Before you started to stretch, you had a very limited and defined number of ways of using these four different sides of yourself. But now you are unbounded in how you will interact and be with everyone. Your world has been blown wide open. Now literally nothing is impossible. You are stretching all day long by the way you are being and your body reflects you being flexible in your life by making you more physically flexible. The connection paves the way.

Humanity has already made
the evolutionary leap.
Critical mass has already occurred.
The whole world is transforming.
Everyone is upgrading.
Everyone's intuition is on fire.

Your Sixth Sense—Intuition

You have learned to stretch in the way you are being all day long. You have both an inside and outside perception of reality that is ever expanding. You are now acknowledging your "sixth sense"—your sixteen types of intuitions in yourself and others. You use your intuition just like you do your eyes, your ears, and your sense of touch. Except your intuition sees without eyes, hears without ears, feels without touching. The intuitions pick up frequencies outside the frequency ranges detectable by your other senses. You see into other people; you hear what is really being said.

You have gained perspective to know what is inside and what is outside yourself. You find yourself using your intuition much more than ever before. It's constantly turned on! You are experiencing synchronicity happening at an increasing rate. You are infinitely more compassionate and empathic.

People now stretch in airports, bus stations, and parks; on sidewalks; in their offices; at the pool and riding stables; at all athletic events; at parties and garage sales; on the TV, in movies, and in plays; on planes, trains, and boats; in the water, in the air, and under the ground; and before, during, and after work, play, sex, and eating. In the near future, it will be very difficult to find anyone who doesn't stretch.

The sum total of all the affects of stretching tells you that you are human, more like every other human than you had realized; but you are also rock, vegetable, animal, and godly. You find yourself revering people for no other reason than simply because they are human. Stretching has taught you that you can enter into the reality of each and every other person—from the inside out! You've learned to acknowledge the Sixteen Geniuses.

⌐

I would never have imagined in a million years,
All the things that have already
happened to me from stretching.
Almost nothing has not changed and
Who I have become is what
I have always wished for.
I can see other people like myself
And in so, treat them as myself.
The Sixteen Geniuses are also within me.

⌐

I respect all your efforts and wish the world to reflect what I know to be possible. I think the world of you.

Resources

Resistance Flexibility Training and the Meridian Flexibility System

www.MeridianStretching.com

Our Web site contains information on the following topics:

- **Resistance Flexibility Training and the Meridian Flexibility System** with on-line streaming videos
- **Studio 16's—the Meridian Stretching Centers** (future complexes include first-floor certified organic restaurant, organic product store, and second-floor Meridian Fitness Studio)
- **Certified Trainers**—locate certified meridian flexibility trainers who offer private sessions and classes near you
- **Resistance flexibility videos**—introduction, intermediate, assisted, and advanced videos; also flexibility videos for most sports

- **News announcements**—Olympic and professional athletes, TV appearances, book tours, magazine articles, and more
- **Online support**—troubleshooting answers when stretching
- **Chat line**—"Talk to Bob"
- **Online real-time private stretching sessions** from anywhere in the world with a certified trainer
- **Workshops and retreats,** including dates and specifics
- **Teacher certificate intensives,** including dates and specifics
- **Meridian fitness equipment and stretching boards**
- **Stretching supplies**—including organic cotton or wool rugs, mats, straps, organic beeswax candles, towels, spring water, and more
- **Organic meridian fitness clothing**—including shorts, T-shirts, socks, sweatshirts, pants, khakis, tops, and more

- **The Total Organic Makeover**—organic foods and supplements: Living Fuel, Garden of Life, First Organics Supplements, olive oil, raw unpasteurized dairy products; organic lifestyle products; towels, blankets, sheets, cleaners, paints, gardening supplies, fasting recommendations, cooking supplies, furniture, refrigeration, transportation, and more
- **Subscription newsletter and information line**—including chat, forum, troubleshooting advice, latest research updates
- **Meridian Teacher Association Hot Line**
- **Special organic sponsors (SOS)**
- **Links to many wonderful organic companies** that offer food, furniture, nontoxic paints, household products, books, music, movies, and more
- **Links to other alternative therapists,** including Dr. Joseph Mercola (Mercola.com)
- **The 16 Geniuses**—sixteen genetic personality types online typing

Organic Resources

The following are wonderful organic companies that—besides being certified organic—have business practices I admire and do incredible things, such as supporting sustainability, fair trade, fair wages, fair distribution of profit, profit sharing, life support and care facilities, donations to nonprofit companies.

Get ready to meet some really great people!

Certified Organic Food

Cascadian Farms
organic frozen fruits and vegetables
719 Melcalf St.
Sedro-Woolley, WA 98284
1-800-624-4123
www.cascadianfarm.com

De Medici Imports
organic olive oil
214 North Main St.
Florida, NY 10921
1-845-651-4400
www.demedici.com

Diamond Organics
next-day fresh organic produce and products
Highway 1
Moss Landing, CA 95039
1-888-674-2642
www.diamondorganics.com

Earthbound Farm
organic fresh salad greens and more
1721 San Juan Highway
San Juan Bautista, CA 95045
1-800-690-3200
www.earthboundfarm.com

Ecofish
environmentally responsible seafood
78 Market St.
Portsmouth, NH 03801
1-603-430-0101
www.ecofish.com

Farmer's Organic Foods

truly free-range eggs

W12599 East Fees Rd.

Alma Center, WI 54611

1-715-964-1317

www.farmersorganicfoods.com

Food for Life

organic sprouted breads

PO Box 1434

Corona, CA 92878

1-800-797-5090

www.foodforlife.com

French Meadow Bakery

organic hemp and other bread

2610 Lyndale Ave.

Minneapolis, MN 55408

1-612-870-4740

www.frenchmeadow.com

Frontier Natural Products

organic spices and herbs

3021 78th St.

Norway, IA 53218

www.frontiercoop.com

Icelandia Natural Sea Salt

60% less sodium, naturally harvested

123 Cloverleaf Lane

Asheville, NC 28803

1-828-277-7564

www.icelandianatural.com

Jimbo's Markets

organic grocery stores

San Diego, Escondido, and Carlsbad, CA

www.jimbos.com

Lundberg Family Farms

organic rice

5370 Church St.

Richvale, CA 95974

1-530-882-4551

www.lundberg.com

McFadden Farm

organic herbs, spices, and more

16000 Powerhouse Rd.

Potter Valley, CA 95469

1-800-544-8320

www.mcfaddenfarm.com

Madhava

agave cactus nectar and natural honey

Lyons, CO

1-303-823-5166

www.madhavahoney.com

Maple Valley

organic maple syrup

919 Front St.

Cashton, WI 54619

1-800-760-1449

www.maplevalleysyrup.com

Olivas de Oro Olive Company

organic olive oil and products

1-866-556-5483

www.olivasdeoro.com

Organic Pastures Dairy Company

organic, raw, unpasteurized,

nonhomogenized dairy products

7221 South Jameson

Fresno, CA 93706

1-877-729-6455

www.organicpastures.com

Petaluma Poultry

organic chicken and turkey

PO Box 7368

Petaluma, CA 94955

1-707-763-1904

www.petalumapoultry.com

Really Raw Honey

truly raw honey products

3500 Boston St., Ste. 32

Baltimore, MD 21224

1-800-732-5729

www.reallyrawhoney.com

Seeds of Change

organic seeds and foods

3250 East 44 St.

Vernon, CA 90058

1-888-762-7333

www.seedsofchange.com

SunRidge Farms

organic dried bulk foods

1055 17th Ave.

Santa Cruz, CA 95062

1-831-462-1280

www.sunridgefarms.com

Trout Lake Farm

organic herbs

PO Box 181

Trout Lake, WA 98650

1-509-395-2025

or

19600 6th St.

Lakeview, CA 92567

1-909-928-6500

www.troutlakefarm.com

Vital Choice Seafood

environmentally responsible seafood

605 30th St.

Anacortes, WA 98221

1-800-608-4825

www.vitalchoice.com

Wholesome Harvest

organic grass-fed meat

RR 1

Colo, IA 50056

1-641-377-3322

www.wholesomeharvest.com

Wild Oats Markets

natural and organic foods

3375 Mitchell Lane

Boulder, CO 80301

1-800-494-9453

www.wildoats.com

Supplements and Remedies

Bach Flower Essences

Bach Flower Remedies
100 Research Dr.
Wilmington, MA 01887
1-800-319-9151
www.nelsonbach.com

Boiron

homeopathic remedies
6 Campus Blvd., Bldg. A
Newtown Square, PA 19073
1-610-325-7464
www.boiron.com

First Organics

certified organic vitamins and supplements
198 East Highway 66
Gallup, NM 87301
1-866-332-9440
www.firstorganics.net

Gaia Herbs

certified organic botanical extracts
108 Island Ford Rd.
Brevard, NC 28712
1-828-884-4242
www.gaiaherbs.com

Garden of Life

supplements and food products
5500 N. Village Blvd., Ste. 202
West Palm Beach, FL 33407
1-561-748-2477
www.gardenoflife.com

Living Fuel

organic, wild-harvested meal replacements,
food bars, and supplements
PO Box 1048
Tampa, FL 33601
1-813-254-5626
www.livingfuel.com

Organic Food Bar

organic food bars
215 E. Organethorpe Ave. #284
Fullerton, CA 92832
1-800-246-4685
www.organicfoodbar.com

Stretch Island Fruit

organic dried fruit
1-360-275-6050
www.stretch-island.com

Sweet Wheat

certified organic wheat grass
PO Box 187
Clearwater, FL 33757
1-888-227-9338
www.sweetwheat.com

Traditional Medicinals

organic teas
PO Box 722345
San Diego, CA 92172
www.tealand.com

Spring Water

Crystal Geyser

mineral waters
55 Francisco St., Ste. 410
San Francisco, CA 94133
1-800-443-9737
www.crystalgeyser.com

Eldorado

natural spring water
PO Box 445
Eldorado Springs, CO 80025
1-303-499-1316
www.eldoradosprings.com

Keeper Springs

protected spring water
96 Spring St.
New York, NY 10012
1-212-925-4544
www.keepersprings.com

Trinity Springs

natural mineral supplement
1101 West River St., Ste. 370
Boise, ID 83702
1-208-433-0867
www.trinitysprings.com

Volvic

natural spring water
1-800-233-6200
www.volvic-na.com

Clothing

American Apparel

organic cotton clothing
747 Warehouse St.
Los Angeles, CA 90021
1-213-488-0226
www.americanapparel.com

Blue Canoe

organic cotton sportswear
PO Box 543
Garberville, CA 95542
1-888-923-1373
www.bluecanoe.com

Cottonfield

organic cotton clothing
PO Box 1386
Brookline, MA 02446
1-888-954-1551
www.cottonfield.com

Earthcreations

earth-dyed organic cotton clothing
3056 Mountainview Way
Bessemer, AL 35020
1-800-792-9868
www.earthcreations.net

Earth Speaks

organic cotton, hemp, and silk clothing
33 Flatbush Ave.
Brooklyn, NY 11217
1-718-797-6898
www.earthspeaks.com

Ecolution
organic cotton and hemp clothing
PO Box 697
Santa Cruz, CA 95061
1-800-973-4367
www.ecolution.com

Hemp Sisters
organic hemp clothing
1210 Chermar Lane
Narberth, PA 19072
1-866-465-4489
www.hemp-sisters.com

Lands Downunder
organic wool clothing and products
212 Foster Ave.
Brooklyn, NY 11230
1-800-790-0332
www.landsdownunder.com

Maggie's Organics
organic cotton clothing and accessories
360 W. Cross St.
Ypsilanti, MI 48197
1-800-609-8593
www.maggiesorganics.com

Organic Cotton Alternatives
organic cotton clothing
3120 Central Ave. SE
Albuquerque, NM 87106
1-888-645-4452
www.organiccottonalts.com

Patagonia
organic cotton clothing
8550 White Fir St.
Reno, NV 89523
1-800-638-6464
www.patagonia.com

Sahara Organics
organic cotton clothing
209 Kearny St.
San Francisco, CA 94108
1-877-472-4272
www.saharaorganics.com

T.S. Designs
nontoxic imprints for clothing
2053 Willow Springs Lane
Burlington, NC 27215
1-336-229-6426
www.tsdesigns.com

Under the Canopy
organic clothing
11421 S. Rogers Circle, Ste. 7
Boca Raton, FL 33487
1-888-226-6799
www.underthecanopy.com

Cosmetics and Body Care

Aubrey Organics
organic shampoos, conditioners, and
cosmetics
4419 N. Manhattan Ave.
Tampa, FL 33614
1-800-282-7394
www.aubrey-organics.com

Dr. Bronner's Magic Soaps

soaps

PO Box 28

Escondido, CA 92033

1-760-743-2211

www.drbronner.com

John Masters Organics

organic shampoos and conditioners

77 Sullivan St.

New York, NY 10012

1-212-343-9590

www.johnmasters.com

Jurlique

holistic skin care and organic cosmetics

2714 Apple Valley Rd. NE

Atlanta, GA 30319

1-404-262-9382

www.jurlique.com

Kiss My Face

organic toothpaste and more

PO Box 224

Gardiner, NH 12525

1-800-262-5477

www.kissmyface.com

Organic Essentials

organic bath products

822 Baldridge St.

O'Donnell, TX 79351

1-800-765-6491

www.organicessentials.com

Rainbow Research

organic hair and skin-care products

170 Wilbur Place

Bohemia, NY 11716

1-800-722-9595

www.rainbowresearch.com

Tom's of Maine

organic toothpaste and more

PO Box 710

Kennebunk, ME 04043

1-800-367-8667

www.tomsofmaine.com

Household Products and Furnishings

Bee Bright Candles

organic honeybee candles

PO Box 411

Santa Cruz, CA 95061

1-831-423-7185

www.beebright.com

Bi-O-Kleen

organic cleaning products

PO Box 820689

Vancouver, WA 98682

1-800-477-0188

www.bi-o-kleen.com

Bioshield Paints

nontoxic paints, floor finishes, cleaners, cork, and more

1330 Rufina Circle

Santa Fe, NM 87507

1-800-621-2591

www.bioshieldpaint.com

Coyuchi
organic cotton sheets, pillowcases,
blankets, towels, and more
PO Box 845
Point Reyes, CA 94956
1-888-418-8847
www.coyuchi.com

Designs for Comfort
Peel Chair and more
1299 Highland Ave.
Needham, MA 02492
1-888-258-2684
www.designsforcomfort.com

Eco Lips
organic lip balms
329 10th Ave. SE
Cedar Rapids, IA 52401
1-866-326-5477
www.ecolips.com

Fire & Light
recycled plates, glassware, vases, and more
45 Ericson Court
Arcata, CA 95521
1-800-844-2223
www.fireandlight.com

Furnature
organic and sustainable furniture
86 Coolidge Ave.
Watertown, MA 02472
1-800-326-4895
www.furnature.com

Heartwood Furniture
sustainable and nontoxic furniture
www.heartwoodindustries.com

Living Tree Paper Company
100% recycled postconsumer paper
1430 Williamette St., Ste. 367
Eugene, OR 97401
1-800-309-2974
www.livingtreepaper.com

Lumiram
full-spectrum lightbulbs
85 Fulton St.
White Plains, NY 10606
1-800-354-5596
www.lumiram.com

Organic Light Photography
photographic prints and cards
www.organiclightphoto.com

Peaceful Valley Farm Supply
organic garden supplies
PO Box 2209
Grass Valley, CA 95945
1-888-784-1722
www.groworganic.com

Preserve
recycled toothbrushes, razors, and more
681 Main St.
Waltham, MA 02451
1-888-354-7296
www.recycline.com

Ringing Mountain Imports

organic and fair trade wool Tibetan rugs

1-888-600-3818

www.ringingmountain.com

Seventh Generation

recycled bathroom products

212 Battery St., Ste. A

Burlington, VT 05401

1-800-456-1191

www.seventhgeneration.com

Spiritual Cinema Circle

spiritual films, books, and CDs

5580 La Jolla Blvd.

La Jolla, CA 92037

1-858-454-3314

www.spiritualcinemacircle.com

Tree of Life

organic cleaning products

405 Golfway West Dr.

St. Augustine, FL 32095

1-904-940-2100

www.treeoflife.com

Via Seating

Swopper Chair

205 Vista Blvd.

Sparks, NV 89434

1-800-433-6614

www.viaseating.com

Zapotec Women's Weaving Cooperative

organic, vegetable-dyed, hand-woven rugs

1-541-745-5690

juanitar@proaxis.com

Organic Organizations

Appetite for a Change organicconsumers .org/sos

BioDemocracy Alliance organic consumers.org/ge-free

BioFach conferences worldwide www .biofach.de

Campaign Against GE Corn organic consumers.org/corn

Clothes for a Change organicconsumers .org/clothes

Coming Clean come-clean.org

GE Free gefreemarkets.org

International Conference on Organic Textiles intercot.org

International Federation of Organic Agriculture Movements ifoam.org

Millions Against Monsanto organic consumers.org/monlink

Monterey Bay Aquarium mbayaq.org

Organic Consumers Association organic consumers.org

Organic Exchange organicexchange.org

Organic Farmers and Gardeners Union organicconsumers.org/ofgu

Organic Trade Association ota.com

Organic Watch organicconsumers.org/ organic

Sustainable Chiapas Program organic consumers.org/chiapas

Recommended Reference Books

Flexibility Training

Devananda, Vishnu Swami. *The Complete Illustrated Book of Yoga*. Three Rivers Press, 1995.

Hewitt, James. *The Complete Yoga Book*. Schocken, 1990.

Iyengar, B.K.S. *Light on Yoga*. Schocken, 1995.

Swenson, David. *Ashtanga Yoga*. Ashtanga Yoga Productions, 1999.

Voss, Dorothy E., Marjorie K. Ionta, and Beverly J. Myers. *Proprioceptive Neuromuscular Facilitation: Patterns and Techniques*. Lippincott Williams and Wilkins, 1985.

Strength Training

Delavier, Frédéric. Strength *Training Anatomy*. Human Kinetics, 2001.

Anatomy and Kinesiology

Netter, Frank H., M.D. *Atlas of Human Anatomy*. Icon Learning Systems, 2002.

Palastanga, Nigel, Derek Field, and Roger Soames. *Anatomy of Human Movement: Structure & Function*. Butterworth-Heinemann, 2002.

Thompson, Clem W., and R. T. Floyd. *Manual of Structural Kinesiology*. McGraw-Hill, 2003.

Traditional Chinese Medicine

Connelly, Dianne M. *Traditional Acupuncture: The Law of the Five Elements*. Traditional Acupuncture Institute, 1994.

Tedeschi, Marc. *Essential Anatomy: For the Healing and Martial Arts*. Weatherhill, 2000.

Teeguarden, Iona Marsaa. *The Joy of Feeling: Bodymind Acupressure*. Japan Publications, 1987.

Personality Type Theory

Arrien, Angeles. *The Tarot Handbook: Practical Applications of Ancient Visual Symbols*. Jeremy P. Tarcher/Putnam, 1997.

Oscar, Ichazo. *The Arican International Journal*. Kent, CT: Arica Institute, 1991.

Riso, Don Richard, and Russ Hudson. *Personality Types: Using the Enneagram for Self-Discovery*. Houghton Mifflin, 1996.

Massage

Biel, Andrew R., and Robin Dorn. *Trail Guide to the Body: How to Locate Muscles, Bones & More!* Books of Discovery, 2001.

Field, Derek. *Anatomy: Palpation and Surface Markings.* Butterworth-Heinemann, 2001.

Nutrition

Balch, Phyllis A., and James F. Balch. *Prescription for Nutritional Healing.* Avery Publishing, 2000.

Fallon, Sally. *Nourishing Traditions: The Cookbook That Challenges Politically Correct Nutrition and the Diet Democrats.* New Trends Publishing, 1999.

Pitchford, Paul. *Healing with Whole Foods: Asian Traditions and Modern Nutrition.* North Atlantic Books, 2002.

Appendix A

The Four Corners of Optimal Nutrition

BY K. C. CRAICHY,
FOUNDER & CEO OF LIVING FUEL, INC.

Even with our current knowledge of nutrition and its impact on health and quality of life, not to mention the ready availability of high-quality foods and supplements, most of us are not meeting our nutritional needs. Consider the stunning prevalence of such diseases as cancer, heart disease, diabetes, and autoimmune disorders. Extensive research has clearly linked such conditions to poor nutrition. Issues such as exposure to toxic chemicals and a high-speed, high-stress lifestyle further complicate these nutritional deficits. The Four Corners of Optimal Nutrition incorporates well-documented but often ignored fundamentals of nutrition and health into one powerful, unified theory.

Corner 1:
Calorie Restriction with Optimal Nutrition (CRON)

CRON diets are known to increase life span by as much as 30 to 50 percent. The key to their success is that they focus not just on calorie-counting, but on consuming high-quality, nutrient-dense foods that deliver a healthy balance of proteins, essential fats, and carbohydrates.

Corner 2:
Low Glycemic Response

The high sugar content in the modern American diet correlates directly to numerous degenerative diseases, from obesity to hypertension to diabetes. A high glycemic (or high sugar) biochemical response is caused by eating foods that rapidly convert to sugar in the bloodstream. Low glycemic foods, by contrast, raise blood sugar levels gradually. They include dark green vegetables, such as broccoli, kale, and spinach, as well as avocados, nuts, and some fruits, such as blueberries and cranberries.

Corner 3: High Antioxidants

Antioxidants are a group of compounds produced by the body that occur naturally in many foods. They protect us from the damage caused by oxidation and its toxic byproducts—free radicals—which can attack and weaken healthy cells, making us more susceptible to disease, and can fast-forward the aging process. One's propensity for illness is directly related to the balance of oxidants to antioxidants within the body. Health protecting antioxidants include tea leaves, berries, apples, onions, and red grapes, as well as supplements of vitamin D and A, vitamin C and full-spectrum vitamin E.

Corner 4: Healthy Fats

Controlled protein intake along with more liberal amounts of healthy fats, such as fish oil, olive oil, and coconut oil, have a very positive effect on health. They increase the fluidity of cell membranes, allowing more nutrients to reach the cells themselves. Healthy fats are found in high concentrations in chia seeds, flax seeds, antioxidant-protected fish oil, borage-seed oil, olives, nuts, coconut, and avocados. These foods also provide critical omega-3 and omega-6 fatty acids that are essential for normal nervous system and brain function.

Foods That Fit the Four Corners

- Fresh, purified, or spring water and caffeine-free teas.
- A variety of salads and green and bright colored, above-ground vegetables—raw, juiced, or slightly steamed.
- Free-range, high-DHA eggs
- Organic chicken or turkey, wild game, grass-fed beef, and fish such as mercury-free pacific salmon, summer flounder, haddock, anchovies, and sardines
- Berries (cranberries, strawberries, raspberries, and blueberries)
- Nuts (almonds, cashews, and macadamias)
- Coconut oil, olive oil, and organic, raw, non-pasteurized dairy products

Avoid sugar and things that turn into sugar quickly, such as snack foods, desserts, soft drinks, sport drinks, coffee, margarine, alcoholic beverages, pasteurized dairy products, unfermented soy products, junk food, fried foods, and foods that are highly refined and processed.

The Science Behind the Meridian Flexibility System

Quantifying Human Range of Motion (QHROM) Research

A six-foot-diameter electromagnetic semi-sphere is projected around the person's body. A 3-D digitizing "wand" is used to touch specific bony landmarks on a person's body to identify his or her x-, y-, z-coordinates. By taking these anthropometric measurements, a 3-D skeleton on the computer is scaled (morphed) to the person's size. As the person moves into sixteen different types of flexibility movements from the Meridian Flexibility System, the skeleton on the computer screen imitates the movements.

The QHROM motion analysis software program graphically displays, records, and analyzes the person's bones rotational interrelationships (BRI) concomitant with these sixteen flexibility movements. Sixteen muscle groups and their ranges of motion are analyzed.

Within fifteen minutes, the computer displays and prints out the person's true flexibility (range of motion, ROM) for all the major joints of the body. The person's flexibility results are displayed numerically and pictorially, and compared to averages, norms, and optimal levels of flexibility.

Individuals can compare the relationships of their bones to ideal models, see to what extent their bones rotate compared to optimal ranges, recognize which muscles are contracting and lengthening to produce their movements, and identify target muscles exhibiting significant limitations in flexibility for the sixteen different stretch movements. Visual comparisons to ideal posture and optimal bone-muscle movement relationships can be studied through an interactive interface.

Targeted areas of significant and potentially dangerous stresses are highlighted. A prioritized list of muscles needing increased flexibility with recommended corrective stretch movements is presented. Reevaluation after treatment can occur at any time, treatment modality accountability assessed, and improvements quantified.

This QHROM system is an extremely accurate and reliable scientific method for diagnosing one's true flexibility. It can be used as a powerful approach for preventing physical injury, planning rehabilitation, improving posture, and evaluating the efficacy of different therapeutic modalities (i.e., changes in ROM through correct practice of the Resistance Flexibility Training techniques can be visually and quantitatively evaluated versus other therapeutic modalities).

It is also one of the best means for helping to optimize athletic performance—by eliminating myofascial malfunctions and stresses. Dara Torres at the 2000 Olympic Games won two gold and three bronze medals, crediting the Meridian Flexibility System and Bob Cooley as significant contributions to her success. Dara brought Bob on *Good Morning America* twice to show America how a thirty-three-year-old woman could be more flexible and faster than she was at sixteen.

In the future, changes in flexibility will be correlated with specific improvements in physiological and psychological health.

Acknowledgments

I'd like to express my gratitude and admiration to the people who continue to contribute so much to so many others' lives:

Pam Mitchell and her family, and the man who was driving the car that struck us.

My family: mother; spirit of my father, sister, and brother; my aunts Carol and Bev; and my masterful Aunt Maxine.

My lifelong partners Tom Longo, Elizabeth Smith Troy, Rose Nataupsky, Lisa Sharkey, Gail Courville, Ann Marie Joyce, Nora Pouillon, Christine Lloreda, and Wendy Graham.

Lyndi Schrecengost, my editor and cowriter, who made writing this first book incredibly enjoyable; Michael Colarito, my photographer; his son James; star organizer Christianna for creating the purely artistic stretching photographs; Graeme Hryniowski for the clear graphics and illustrations; Christine Lloreda for her trustworthy and caring support always; Trish Todd and Nancy Hancock, my editors at Simon & Schuster, for their interest in my manuscript from the beginning; my agent, Michael Broussard, whom I call the talent magnet; Einsenberg associates for wonderful graphics for the stretch photos; much love to Joni Evans and Mel Berger of the William Morris Agency; Jill Lieber of *USA Today*; Debbie and Arielle Ford; K. C. Craichy for writing Appendix A on nutrition and Nora Pouillon for writing the foods for the seasons chapter; Ira Gubernick, my peaceful and communicative lawyer; Olympic gold medal swimmer Dara Torres for showing the world what being more flexible can do for anyone at any age.

My closest friends Matt Bulanger, Diane Tarantino, Brian Clague, Nica Faulkner, Wendy Graham, Chris Maher, Steve Hoffman, Marcus Riggleman, Steve Sierra, Gerry and Jackie Reese, Nic Bartol-

Iota, Johnny Blackburn, Barbara Chandler, Nancy Melon, Mark Sweeney, Jesse Cool, Liz Koch Oberdorffer, Joanna Direndre, Phoebe Barnes, Bjorn Holtan, Teresa Iacovino, John Amaral, Sue Stenger, Sally Jackson, David Levitt, Dave Allen, Michelle Kessler, Nancy Heszelton, Dierdre Morris, Prudence Whittlesey, Ann Marie Lupacchino, Scott and Katherine Eibel and son, Rebecca Marston, Marybeth and Jeff Randall, Dan, Elaine Harrington, Peter Johanson, Suzanne Cavedon, Marylyn Smith, Madeleine Smith Troy, Bruce Hale, Doran Christie, Jonathan and Michelle Kalman, Scott and Maryanne Reese, Drayton Bowles, Prince Albert, Bruno, and Karl Karlson.

All my Boston, New York, Pennsylvania, Florida, and California friends who stretch: Doug, Casey, and Greg Gleicher; John MacDonald; Michael Mac Donald, Danny Pelzig; Kerry Troy; Kerry and Sean Sheeran; Alan, Allene, and Jacob Fisch; Sharon Blumenthaul; Ritu Gorczyca; Robin Garstka and her newborn; Patrick Barry; Ann Whittaker; Michelle Kessler; George Deptula; Nick Love; Aaron Sugarman and his partner Tammy; Steve Knapp; Jim Rushford; Nora and Suzanne Smith; Amber Flynn and Gary Crowley; Ed Coakley; Pat Kirk; Jennifer Kent and her brother, Roberto Perez; Evelyn Clark; Corey; Henry Nye; Roy Iggeleton; Rush; Scott; and Ike.

My extended family: Carol and Gill Maghakian, and "Bro" Longo.

Athletes and coaches: Allan Houston, Eric Flaim, Rob Herb, Eli Fairfield, Sean Scott, Albert Hanneman, Billy Kheir, Nicholas Roby, Alyssa Carlson, and Whitney.

All the certified meridian flexibility interns and the people who stretch with them.

Heroines and heroes: Janet Travel, Sister Kenny.

My generous sponsors: Living Fuel, Maggie's Organic Clothing, Earthbound Farms, Oliva de Oro, Coyuchi Organic Cotton Bedding, Stretch Island Fruit, Earthspeaks.

Organic pioneers Nora Poullion, Bena Burda, Katherine Demotto, Eric Henry, James Vreeland, Eric and son, K. C. Craichy, Mark McAfee.

All the people who were photographed for the stretches: Ben and Andy Hoff, Nic Bartollota, Thomas Bakalars, Katie Thomas, Johnny Blackburn, Tom Longo, Mark Sweeney, Robin Garstka, Nancy Heselton, Barbara Chandler, Edith Keller, Josh Rilla, Ann Marie Joyce, Bjorn Holtan, Matt Belanger, Frank Albanese, Elizabeth Troy, Dustin Avol, Robert King, Christopher Maher, Suzanne Cavedon, Marcus Riggleman, Joanna DiRice, William Rios, Carolyn Sheean, James Colavito, James Warren, Nino DeAngelis and Scott Do for hairstyling, Russ.

Health-care providers: Mary Maloney, Dr. David Simon, Dr. Karl Maret, and Dr. Joseph Mercola.

And to all the angels protecting others and myself.

Index

Page numbers in *italics* refer to illustrations.

About the Author

BOB COOLEY is the founder and president of the Meridian Stretching Centers and the developer of Resistance Flexibility Training. An expert on flexibility and its relation to health, his theories unite biomechanics, structural kinesiology, Hatha yoga, Traditional Chinese Medicine, and the Sixteen Geniuses (a genetically based personality system) into his powerful stretching program, The Meridian Flexibility System™.

Bob has more than twenty years of teaching and research experience in such diverse fields as biomechanics, motor learning, flexibility and strength training, movement, Chinese Medicine, personality types, and psychology. In 1978, he addressed the U.S. Olympic Swim Committee's Advanced Coaches Seminar on his head-up free-style swim stroke, which he developed to avoid "swimmer's shoulder" and as the fastest way to swim freestyle. In 1979, he wrote a paper with Dorothy Voss, one of the developers of PNF, which was the forerunner of current rehabilitative PNF stretching techniques. Bob did graduate study at the University of Massachusetts Exercise Science Department, where he worked with the developer of current biomechanical computer analysis, and at the University of Maryland Biophysical Studies Department.

Bob has stretched Dara Torres, Olympic gold medalist swimmer; Eric Flaim, three-time Olympic speed skater; Prince Albert of Monaco; Allan Houston of the New York Knicks; Jayson Werth of the Los Angeles Dodgers; Daniel Pelzig, choreographer for the Boston Ballet; athletes from the Boston Bruins; and professional dancers. He is currently a flexibility and psychological trainer for professional and Olympic athletes, severely injured individuals, and CEOs. He has appeared on *Good Morning America* and Fox and in *Sports Illustrated*, *Self*, and *Outside* magazines.